A
CQI SYSTEM
FOR
HEALTHCARE

How The Williamsport Hospital Brings Quality to Life

Tim Mannello

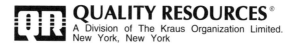

QUALITY RESOURCES®
A Division of The Kraus Organization Limited.
New York, New York

Most Quality Resources books are available at quantity discounts when purchased in bulk. For more information contact:

Special Sales Department
Quality Resources
A Division of The Kraus Organization Limited
902 Broadway
New York, New York 10010
800-247-8519

Printed in the United States of America

97 96 95   10 9 8 7 6 5 4 3 2 1

Quality Resources
A Division of The Kraus Organization Limited
902 Broadway
New York, New York 10010
800-247-8519

∞

The paper used in this publication meets the minimum requirements of American National Standard for Information Sciences—Permanence of Paper for Printed Library Materials, ANSI Z39.48-1984.

ISBN 0-527-76290-3

Library of Congress Cataloging-in-Publication Data
Mannello, Timothy.
    A CQI system for healthcare : how the Williamsport Hospital brings quality to life / Timothy Mannello.
        p.   cm.
    Includes index.
    ISBN 0-527-76290-3 (hardcover)
    1. Hospital care—Quality control.   2. Total quality management.
3. Williamsport Hospital (Williamsport, Pa.)   4. Hospital care—Quality control—Case studies.   I. Title.
    [DNLM: 1. Williamsport Hospital (Williamsport, Pa.)   2. Total Quality Management—organization & administration—Pennsylvania.
3. Delivery of Health Care—organization & administration —Pennsylvania.   4. Hospital Administration—Pennsylvania.   WX 28 AP4 M2c 1995]
    RA972.M345   1995
362.1'1'0685—dc20
DNLM/DLC
for Library of Congress   94-46508
                                                                          CIP

To Gisella and Albert, my Mother and Father, who like Winston Churchill were "easily satisfied with the best."

CONTENTS

Foreword

The central thesis of this book—that hospitals, as service organizations, have a moral and ethical obligation not only to meet but to exceed the expectations of those they serve—may strike some as obvious when they consider their own quality improvement mission, which may articulate a similar premise.

As you begin this book, however, it is important for you to understand that the success of the *process* at The Williamsport Hospital & Medical Center is underpinned by the fundamental belief that the ultimate success of any quality initiative is directly dependent upon the inculcation of a quality *culture* throughout the organization. The establishment of that culture cannot happen as the result of a board action or corporate directive. Rather, it must be founded on a belief that people aspire to excel and are nurtured by an environment that supports personal growth and development, sustains a commitment to continuous system improvements, and is supported by institutional policies and objectives that allow all constituencies within the hospital family to recognize the commitment to quality as the cultural essence of the organization. That is when a quality effort makes the transition from a *program*—that is often seen by others as "the management fad of the week"—to an organizational *process* that is believed and supported by those who must live it, if it is to produce the demonstrable results that each of us seek.

A CQI System for Healthcare is not another collection of worn out, business school axioms and wisdom, but is an extraordinary treasure chest of information that you can apply in *your* organization if you perceive quality, not as a program, but as a cultural process.

As I sit down to write this foreword, we are fast approaching the end of another year and look forward with much anticipation to January, the beginning of a new year. Janus, you may recall, was the Roman god of doors and gateways and, hence, of beginnings and endings. He is usually pictured with two faces looking in opposite directions—one old, looking back on the year just ended and one young, looking forward to the year ahead. Like Janus, I look back with pride on the last decade and the growth of the quality process here at The Williamsport Hospital & Medical Center. Ten years ago, we embarked on a continuous quality improvement initiative that would improve the quality of our services and the process by which those services were delivered while, at the same time, exemplifying an empathetic and compassionate approach to the delivery of care. That commitment culminated in the selection of the hospital as the 1993 recipient of healthcare's most prestigious honor, the Healthcare Forum's "Commitment to Quality Award."

I also look forward to the challenges that lie ahead as healthcare faces unprecedented change. That change offers a unique opportunity to redefine our place in a reformed environment. Providers are feeling both elated and apprehensive. On the one hand we are gratified that America has finally acknowledged what we have known for years (that the healthcare system needs serious attention). On the other hand, we are concerned about what national reform initiatives may ultimately mean for our communities and the patients we serve. Williamsport, Pennsylvania chose not to wait for national forces to reshape the delivery system. Instead, we responded by forming the Susquehanna Health System, an organization consisting of The Williamsport Hospital & Medical Center, Divine Providence Hospital, Muncy Valley Hospital, Susquehanna Physician Services (a multi-specialty physician group employing more than 100 physicians in more than 30 practice locations), Susquehanna Regional Home Health Services, and a variety of other organizations in support of a single vision: *to make this community the healthiest community in the United States.* An integral part of that new commitment will be the System's quality process as we seek to form a fully integrated delivery network that will go beyond treating the sick and the injured to assume responsibility for managing the care of the population and the communities we serve and, ultimately, improve health status.

As we look forward to the challenges that lie ahead, I am greatly comforted in the realization that a fundamental quality culture and *process* exist within the Susquehanna Health System that will allow us to succeed in a rapidly changing healthcare environment, and I am grateful that Tim Mannello will remain a leading architect of and our evangelist to that process.

Donald R. Creamer
President, CEO
Susquehanna Health System

Acknowledgments

This book is the story of the achievement of an extraordinary group of people: The Williamsport Hospital & Medical Center's board of managers and corporate staff who have consistently developed and overseen the implementation of the Hospital's effective strategic plans; our department heads and supervisors who, in their capacity as team builders and service managers, have enabled and motivated our employees to work together in giving their best to our patients and other customers; and our employees, physicians, volunteers, and auxilians who have made "Go-Beyond Service" a tradition here at The Williamsport Hospital & Medical Center. I thank them all for giving me such a wonderful story to tell.

The Williamsport Hospital & Medical Center's story would never have been told without Debbie Loner. Night-after-night, weekend-after-weekend over the course of a full year, Deb gave up her free time to type the innumerable drafts and to provide all of the time-consuming logistical work needed to support the publication of this book. Jen Mitchell and Toni Hiller backed Debbie up to ensure we never missed our production deadlines. The story would not have been told as well as it is without the generously offered sound advice of my editor at Quality Resources, Cindy Tokumitsu; the entire staff at Quality Resources, especially Mike Sinocchi, the managing editor; the external reviewer, Ned Barber; my "quality soul brother," Bill McClain, vice president of marketing and The Williamsport Hospital & Medical Center's corporate "wordsmith"; and Mike Scherneck, who proofed the text. I thank them all for making this a better book.

This book will probably be published about the time when my next performance evaluation is due. Consequently, I would like to acknowledge my wonderful boss, Don Creamer, for leading and sustaining The Williamsport Hospital & Medical Center's decade-long pursuit of quality. Seriously, the pace of the pack is set by the speed of its leader. Don's "let's do it" attitude and sure-footed sense of direction have fostered a self-reliant can-do mind-set among my colleagues on the Hospital's corporate staff: Steve Johnson, our chief operating officer, who has helped make quality and operations inseparable; Jeannie Hill, our vice president of nursing and Candy Dewar, our assistant vice president of nursing, who have worked with Patient Care Managers to integrate our nursing quality initiatives into our hospital-wide quality efforts; Mike Scherneck, our vice president for fiscal affairs, who has helped us maintain an employee/patient-focused, moral sense of profit; Bill McClain, our vice president for marketing, whose influence has guided us in maintaining an outside/in, customer-driven service ethic; Jack Bustin, our vice president for business development, who has recommended business opportunities that coincide with customer needs and our ability to do a superior job; Joe English, M.D., our house champion for the very best in health care for our patients; and Maureen Karstetter, our Foundation Director who is a model for CQI involvement through her active involvement in the work of our CQI Teams.

Don Creamer, Steve Johnson, Bill McClain, Bob Ireland, and Bob Wallace contributed substantially to the resources contained in this book and, together with the other members of our MEDIMPROVE Committee, to the conceptualization and execution of CQI at The Williamsport Hospital & Medical Center. So have many others: there were our Cycle of Service team leaders, such as Tom Schnars, Mark Grace, Denise Clark, Mary Chancellor, Bob Kane, Jim Huebert, Rhona Wilk, Kim Fisher, and Roseanne Mattiace. There were top-flight department heads who have reported to me over the last 10 years: Rita Spangler, Dave Heiney, Kathy Allen, Charlie Wolverton, Joyce Wise and Dick Landis; Mike Heyd and Conrad Shull from our Learning Resource Center; the wonderful employees, especially our 240 C.A.R.E. Employees of the Month; and there were many others too numerous to mention.

Our county—Lycoming County—is blessed with an outstandingly talented Medical Staff led by effective presidents of our Medical Staff over the last decade (Ralph Kaiser, M.D., Wallace Bednarz, M.D., Randall Hipple, M.D., Glen Hofstrom, M.D., and Tim Pagana, M.D.). Our Medical Staff has scored in the superior range in several independent national studies. Other members, such as Earl Miller, M.D., Marcia

Finn, M.D., Dave Finn, M.D., Greg Frailey, M.D., Adel Messeih, M.D., Tim Pagana, M.D., Terry Belles, M.D., Don Leathers, M.D., John Burks, M.D., Jeff Verzella, M.D., Warren Robinson, M.D., Claude Williams, M.D., Keith Shenberger, M.D., Don Nardone, M.D., and Jeff Wetstone, M.D., and other Family Practice Residents have loaned their considerable talents to our CQI efforts over the years.

Now that we have formed an Alliance with our former competitors, Divine Providence Hospital and Muncy Valley Hospital, we look forward to an even more successful quality effort as part of the Susquehanna Health System (SHS). For what is yet to come, I thank visionary Board leaders like Dick DeWald, Dean Fisher, Ralph Nardi, and Birch Phillips who, together with Don Creamer, Sister Jean Mohl, and Kirby Smith, pioneered the establishment of SHS. Thanks to the dedicated and caring managers, employees, physicians, volunteers, and Auxilians of our new partner hospitals—we are now in a position together to provide high-quality, cost-effective, accessible, and compassionate care to the communities we serve.

Finally, a sincere "thank you" to my mother and father, my brother, Sammy, his wife, Barb, and to my sister, Mary Ann, and her husband, Frank—all of whose work has influenced me because it has always been characterized by this belief: "If you can't do it right, don't do it at all." And, sincere thanks to my wife, Kathy, my son Sean, and Esther, Ann, Miss Jessie, and Tripper who have made our home a warm and inviting haven for a fledgling writer.

Introduction

A truly great hospital is a hospital in which
extremely small things are done extraordinarily well by
virtually everybody almost all of the time.

In *And the Band Played On,* Randy Shilts documented the ominous statistics accumulated in the early 1980s on the introduction, spread, and devastation of AIDS in the United States. Despite the growing scientific evidence, attention to AIDS was scant, governmental funding for AIDS research and education was negligible, and the identification of heterosexual mainstream Americans with AIDS was virtually non-existent.

In 1985, Rock Hudson developed and soon died from AIDS. Then, we saw the human story of one person in before-and-after pictures of the star, in old movies co-starring Doris Day, and in their last meetings on the evening news. Suddenly, newspaper and magazine stories and TV newscasts and documentaries covered the phenomenon with growing frequency and in great depth. What a mountain of statistics failed to draw attention to, a single, vivid, widely seen personal story brought to the consciousness of Americans from coast to coast.

There is a great lesson here for making quality happen in American businesses. "Popular introduction," Bertrand Russell, the philosopher, once said, "depends upon the emotional interest of the instances, not upon their number." People are moved to action by vivid images— images that are concrete, tangible, and spatially and temporally set. Joseph Stalin put it this way: "The death of a single Russian soldier is a tragedy. A million deaths is a statistic." The degree to which quality messages excite and motivate people to act rather than merely understand is directly correlated to the vividness with which the message is conveyed.

Because my purpose in this book is to energize people to implement quality, not merely think about it, I have chosen the story, the illustration, and the anecdote as my principal assistants. No one I know ever fell passionately in love with a standard deviation. Some who read about the real live exemplars of quality portrayed in this book will, I hope, find a warm spot in their heart for the appreciative smile and effusive gratitude of a customer who has experienced go-beyond quality service.

In the mid-1960s, the Senate Intelligence Committee reported that about 85 percent of the most valuable information needed by the Central Intelligence Agency could be found in foreign newspapers, books, and published government reports. What was needed, the committee concluded, was more analysis and use of readily available information—not more spies.

Despite this wise advice, the unraveling of the U.S.S.R. and the Eastern Bloc Communist countries that began in August 1989, came as a surprise to the American intelligence community. The signs had been clear for years that the European Communist economies were on the verge of collapse. Nevertheless, aside from a few magazines like the *National Review,* the media—and our government—scrambled for explanations when these decaying economies fomented the thunderous collapse of their political sponsors.

On a far less global scale, something similar is going on among many U.S. companies currently launching new continuous quality improvement efforts. Too often, many of their leaders have embarked on a quest for the Holy Grail, the Lost Ark, the genie in the bottle, the silver bullet—the inside secret to quality success. Somehow, they ended up digging for precious stones in the basements of jewelry stores. Soon after, like luckless prospectors, they've given up their pursuit and declared their flirtation with quality improvement a rendezvous with a tantalizing but ultimately unfulfilling fad. Undoubtedly they are off, yet again, to romancing other stones.

We at The Williamsport Hospital & Medical Center avoided this pitfall when we began our continuous quality improvement (CQI) odyssey almost a decade ago. Since then, we have found an abundance of information in the available literature about conceptualizing and implementing CQI initiatives. Some of it was good; some of it, bad. Much of it was repetitive. But we put things together in ways that suited our customers and ourselves. We plugged away at inspiring, motivating, and enabling our employees to make quality a daily habit.

And, violà—wonder of wonders—our customers and our employees said it was good and the Healthcare Forum and Witt Associates named The Williamsport Hospital & Medical Center the National Commitment to Quality Award winner for 1993.

So we decided to write a book in which we could share our quality ideas, ideals, implementation strategies, and resources with the modest hope that some of what worked for us might, in some adapted form, help readers like you as well.

1

Quality Rules at The Williamsport Hospital & Medical Center

"The customer is our boss. Quality is our work.
Value for the money is our goal."

—Mars, Inc.

It all started with the answer to a simple question at one of the first meetings of The Williamsport Hospital & Medical Center's corporate staff more than 10 years ago. Toward the end of the meeting, our president and CEO Don Creamer said, "Several people have suggested we create a position for a patient representative. What do you think?" Our vice-president of marketing, Bill McClain immediately chimed in, "No single employee should be our hospital's patient representative. *We all should be the patients' representatives.*" Every one of us, including Don, agreed with Bill. With that anchoring belief, our quality journey began.

At a time when the prevailing mood about quality was, "If it ain't new, it can't be true," we at The Williamsport Hospital & Medical Center reminded ourselves that creativity is as much looking at existing but unapplied models in innovative ways as it is thinking up entirely new ones. We'd soon craft a more eloquent version of the goal of CQI when we developed our first corporate objective. At this point, however, we began with a seminal conviction: the best thing we could do for the financial success of the institution and for the personal and professional fulfillment of our employees was to do a bang-up job for our patients and our other customers. Instead of joining the paradigm-bashing

1

bandwagon, we eclectically selected from already successful but widely untried quality paradigms—the ones that made Tom Peters and Karl Albrecht, among others, quality gurus; Karl Jarslen of Scandinavian Airlines and Fred Smith of Federal Express, among others, quality trailblazers; and companies as large as Disney World and as small as Stew Leonard's Dairy, among others, quality legends unmatched anywhere in the world.

Adherence to this old-time quality religion has helped us achieve what Mark H. McCormack calls, in *What They Didn't Teach You at Harvard Business School* (Bantam, 1984), the forgotten and untaught goals of business: maintaining old customers, creating new customers, and making it easy for our customers to do business with us. Even more, it has helped our business become a better place for employees to work and has contributed mightily to our superior financial performance that has been documented in independent comparative studies done by Coopers & Lybrand.

Service companies of all kinds—retailers, banks, hotels, hospitals, or airlines—that are really serious about quality live by certain beliefs. How do we know? Being a student is a permanent way of life for managers at The Williamsport Hospital & Medical Center. Five of our corporate officers completed their master's degrees in the last 10 years. One of our colleagues has two master's degrees. Two years ago, a corporate officer with a master's degree passed state boards as a registered nurse. All corporate officers are Master's prepared and all are voracious readers in their professional fields. Many of the quality initiatives at The Williamsport Hospital & Medical Center were sparked by our understanding of the principles as they are reflected in the select bibliography that concludes this book.

The kind of service excellence at The Williamsport Hospital & Medical Center is a possibility for many service companies. That's because the most basic distinction between quality service winners and also-rans stems from a demonstrable difference in corporate attitude more than from a measurable difference in corporate aptitude. Companies that succeed in progressing toward customer value improvement live by a quality creed that makes them readily recognizable—a creed that we've seen take root, flower, and flourish in a small unpretentious town known to outsiders only as the home of Little League Baseball.

The tenets of the creed we try to live by are as simple to state as they are difficult to emulate. They turn out to be similar to the beliefs described in *Built to Last: Successful Habits of Visionary Companies* by James C. Collins and Jerry I. Porras (Harper Collins, 1994) and in *The Race Without a Finish: Lessons From Malcolm Baldrige Award Winners* by Warren H. Schmidt and Jerome P. Finnigan (Jossey-Bass, 1992). The rest of this chapter explains the tenets of this creed as we've come to learn and practice them.

QUALITY RULE 1: Quality Is Our Business

The first decision we made about quality at The Williamsport Hospital & Medical Center was that quality healthcare was our business and that quality was and will always be everyone's one and only job. With us, quality is not *extra* work, it *is* the work. Our strategic plan embraced the conclusions of the Profit Impact Measurement Studies (PIMS), which indicated that quality is unquestionably the competitive edge in virtually every sort of manufacturing and service business.

So, we defined our mission and corporate value statement in quality terms:

- Mission Statement: The Williamsport Hospital & Medical Center has a long-standing commitment to provide quality services to the people of north central Pennsylvania and to manage the process by which quality care is delivered.
- Corporate Value: Continuously demonstrate the highest regard for the two most important groups of people in our enterprise: our employees and our customers.

Next, we developed corporate goals that were quality goals. In their abbreviated form, they are:

- Goal 1: Deliver go-beyond quality and value that surpass customer expectations for personal service, user-friendly systems, and favorable healthcare outcomes and processes through a three-pronged continuous quality improvement strategy: C.A.R.E., TQM, and MEDIMPROVE.

3

- Goal 2: Enlist our employees' unified pursuit of continuous quality during every moment of truth (i.e., those employee-customer encounters when customers evaluate how good a service is).
- Goal 3: Provide high-quality services at competitive prices.
- Goal 4: Increase the hospital's market share.
- Goal 5: Improve and strengthen the hospital's relationship with its defined medical staff.

By requiring all of our operational plans to derive from these guiding principles, we set out to ensure that we would never deviate from a relentless preoccupation with service excellence. We repeated our long-term commitment over and over again in many ways including this personal story:

> Once as I walked toward the express lane of a supermarket, I was preceded by a woman carrying a bottle of Coca-Cola. A well-dressed VIP type stepped in front of her with a cart overflowing with groceries. Throughout the long check-out period, the old woman maintained her kind and patient smile. When it was finally her turn, the old woman reached over to pay for her Coke. I'll never forget what the clerk said to her, "Don't worry about paying for the Coke, Ma'am. I put it on the hot-shot's bill."

We think that quality companies need heroes, and the old woman in this story is one of our favorites. She's our patron saint, the perfect model of "stick-to-it-iveness." Service businesses aren't likely to become their best selves without a single-minded, unflagging and unfailing dedication to, and execution of, world-class quality. Like the woman in our story, quality-minded companies need to be patient. In *Quality Progress,* David W. Hutton states, "The leading companies are not necessarily the ones that made the best start or are using the most advanced methodologies. They are those who have simply kept at it."

QUALITY RULE 2: Treat Your Customers Like Gold

From the outset of our CQI efforts almost a decade ago, our hospital has been a market-driven institution. Our CEO's academic background is in marketing, and we have strongly emphasized being an outside-in rather than an inside-out organization. To us, that means making our customers—our patients first and foremost, their families and friends, our guests, our physicians, our payors and our community—the be-all and end-all of everything we do. We do so because we are firm believers in the moral of the following story that really hits home with everyone in Williamsport, the birthplace of Little League Baseball, the home of the Little League World Series, and a community in love with America's favorite pastime:

> Three umpires were arguing about what it meant to be an umpire. The first said, "There are balls and there are strikes, and we call them the way they are." The second objected, "No, no, no. There are balls and there are strikes, and we call them the way we see them." The third umpire, one who had been at it for many years, set them both straight, "You've got it all wrong," he said. "There are balls and there are strikes, but they ain't nothin' till we call them."

No question in our minds, the customers call the game. They are the umpires, the final arbiters of service quality. As quality expert Karl Albrecht puts it, "The single most important measure of the quality of the service is the service quality as perceived by our customers compared to our competitors." Front and center, at the initial conceptualization of every quality project and at its concluding evaluation are customers and the service expectations they bring to the service experience.

Customers bring two key requirements to every service encounter: they have a problem they want solved, and they want a good experience. They want what's wrong to be fixed, and they want to be treated right. In a healthcare setting, that comes down to a favorable healthcare outcome provided in accordance with the highest standards of *c*ourtesy, *a*ttentiveness, *r*esponsiveness, and *e*mpathy—in a word, with C.A.R.E.

In *Delivering Quality Service* (The Free Press, 1990), Valerie Zeithaml and her co-authors report research about customer expectations that coincides with our experience. Customers, they say, expect service providers to:

- Be good, to aim at getting it right the first time (reliability—an important nuance about this one later).

5

- Look good in every way from the aesthetics of their service setting, their dress and grooming, to the genuineness and professionalism of their communication, especially their nonverbal communication.
- Embody and project dependability and trustworthiness (assurance).
- Serve as their problem solver or, that failing, find them a problem-solver—saying, in effect, "I'll fix it or if I can't, I'll help you find someone who can" (responsiveness).
- Treat them the way they'd like to be treated in similar circumstances (empathy).

This basic advice about customer focus often gets overlooked in practice. In their combined 38 original points, Joseph Juran, Philip Crosby, and W. Edwards Deming never once mention the word *customer*—never once! As Karl Albrecht observes: "Too many quality initiatives start by measuring and counting tangible work products and processes without any evidence that improving them would contribute to the ultimate success of the business or the satisfaction of the customer (*Modern Healthcare,* Jan. 4, 1993)."

What separates the walkers from the talkers? Unquestionably, an actual—as opposed to simply rhetorical—fixation on customers and their current, real expectations. A University of Wisconsin study reported in the April 1991 issue of *The Economist* drew this conclusion: "The extent to which an organization maintains a *customer* focus determines the difference between quality efforts that fail and quality efforts that succeed."

Success depends not on the proliferation of self-managing CQI teams, not on the sophistication of analytical process tools, not on the diversity and complexity of one's statistical repertoire—but on the accurate, up-to-date understanding of customers and their expectations. Your customer—the buck starts here. Not a bad twist on Truman for the seriously quality-minded.

QUALITY RULE 3: Concentrate CQI Efforts Only on Extremely Important Customer Requirements

A popular saying at our hospital 10 years ago used to be, "Leaders make sure organizations do things the *right way*." We translated that

6

insight into an executive obligation to ensure that we selected the right things—the very highest customer identified priorities—as the exclusive targets of our CQI efforts. At that time, we knew instinctively what the 1992 International Quality Study demonstrated empirically: "The best performers are able to distinguish the extremely *important* imperatives from the mass of important imperatives and then to concentrate extra energy and resources on a handful of differentiating factors."

"Busyness," we decided, was not our business. That meant we would truly have to understand the world of the customer. The world of quality begins to make sense once you clearly see the face and know the mind of your customers so well that you understand their most important expectations. Not just *all* their important unmet expectations, but their *very most* important unmet expectations. There's a difference. In our hospital's emergency room, the physician encounter is important. The nurse encounter is important, too. But for our customers, the receptionist encounter turned out to be the most important encounter of all. Making that encounter all that it needed to be improved our customers' ratings of us dramatically.

Companies that take their customer seriously have enjoyed substantial pay-offs. Until recently, American sneaker manufacturers had not been able to penetrate the Japanese market. That is, until New Balance did so several years ago. How? By altering their production process at great expense to accommodate the generally much shorter length and broader width of Japanese feet and by branching into colors like gold and black, which are more popular among Japanese consumers than Americans. The result: more than a million Japanese now wear New Balance sneakers.

An Australian drugstore chain discovered that their customers' highest unrealized priority was easy and confidential access to the pharmacist. This pharmacy chain has embarked on a five-year renovation program to transform its drug stores into customer-friendly professional places of business that will allow customers the privacy they desire with their pharmacists.

The Australian drugstore chain and New Balance encouraged their customers to actually define their business. In Albrecht's terms, they brought the power of the customer into the center of their businesses. Early on, we thought this approach provided a formula for success. We embraced it and set out to make it happen.

7

The Williamsport Hospital & Medical Center's findings on our patients' high-priority expectations coincide with results of studies published in the past five years. Our patients base their decisions to return to us and to recommend us to others for care on:

- The cheerfulness of our hospital's staff and atmosphere.
- Employee sensitivity to the inconvenience caused by the customer's hospitalization.
- Staff members' and especially nurses' keeping them well informed about the medical tests they receive.
- The provision of adequate information and explanations to patients and their families.
- Staff members' and again especially nurses' attentiveness to their special needs.
- The caring behaviors, sensitive attitudes, and empathy of all of our employees and volunteers.

Much of our intensive training and supervisory attention has been concentrated on ensuring that these attitudes and behaviors are present in a go-beyond fashion during each key moment of truth. We're sure this effort has paid off. Over the last five years, 99.8 percent of our patients tell us they would return for services and recommend us to others.

QUALITY RULE 4: Deliver Go-Beyond Quality

So you have a solid fix on your customers' most important imperatives. Now what? Merely satisfying them, we thought, would make us also-rans. We became intrigued with what Ken Blanchard later called legendary service and Anderson and Zemke called knock-your-socks-off service. We called it go-beyond service. This book describes it in detail. To provide a parallel example from outside healthcare based on an experience we all know and love:

There's this extraordinary gas station in California called Chevron North. It's right across the street from another gas station. A businessman leaving a nearby airport two years ago reported what he called a typical customer experience there. As he approached, he noticed that gas at Chevron North's competitor was 50 cents a gallon cheaper but that Chevron North's lot was loaded with cars and the other gas station was empty. He was fascinated by the unexpected contrast. So, he pulled his car into Chevron North. It didn't take him long to find out why. As he pulled up to the gas pump, three well-dressed attendants came up to his car and asked him if he would be kind enough to release the hood and step out of the car. They then efficiently checked his brake fluid, his windshield wiper fluid, the volume and concentration of his radiator coolant, his oil, his battery, and the belts. They took out and cleaned the air filter with a compressed air gun and inflated the four tires to the right pressure. Next, they washed and dried his windshield inside and out, vacuumed the interior, cleaned his ashtrays, and asked if he would like them to tidy-up his glove compartment and his trunk. After they returned him to the driver's seat, they asked him if he would like coffee or tea (caffeinated or decaffeinated; with or without sugar or artificial sweetener) or soda (diet or regular). They gave him a copy of *USA Today* and, when they had filled his tank and concluded the credit card transaction, they bid him farewell and handed him a card that read: "We sell gas, too."

That's what we call go-beyond quality—transforming a moment of truth into a magic moment. A moment of truth is an encounter between a customer and an employee during which the customer makes a judgment about the quality of a service. A *Magic moment* is a pivotal moment of truth during which an employee exceeds the expectations of the customer for the contact and transforms the moment into a unique and memorable experience. At go-beyond businesses, employees do not merely meet the customer's basic needs. They don't merely satisfy their expectations or desires. In go-beyond businesses, employees surprise the customer with the unexpected so that they gain a special place in the customer's heart. In these businesses, discretionary effort is the norm, not the exception.

In the September/October 1993 issue of *The Healthcare Forum,* David O. Weber described three of the almost 10,000 magic moments honored so far at our hospital:

"For the child who'd been struck by a car, it was the arrival of paramedic Michael Matzinger on the pediatric floor the next afternoon with a new outfit (bought on his day off) to replace the ragged but prized 'school clothes' he'd had to scissor off the protesting boy in the ambulance."

"For the pregnant teenager alone and in labor, it was the unflagging company of family planning counselor Billie Stone, who remained by her side for 12 hours—on her own time—to see the baby born."

"For the 93-year old man convalescing in a nursing home, it was an outing to his beloved mountain cabin for Christmas dinner cooked on a old coal stove by family practice resident, Jonathan Chu, M.D. Dr. Chu had bought the groceries and driven the man to the cabin after a full day and night on hospital duty, to fulfill a reassurance he'd given the elderly patient at discharge a week earlier."

Exciting quality means creating good surprises like these for the customer. But, to all of us at The Williamsport Hospital & Medical Center, it means more than that. As we have seen in the O.J. Simpson case, a single destructive event can forever shatter a sparkling public image. It takes only one cloud to eclipse the sun. So, too, a bad surprise in a single moment of truth can overshadow all of the magic moments experienced by a patient throughout an entire cycle of service. Recently, a gentleman came to me with a complaint. His wife had had a long inpatient stay and was receiving outpatient treatment. He said that everyone had treated them well. There were no hassles or delays. His wife had responded remarkably well to her treatment. Everything had gone perfectly—until the night before, when in the course of describing his wife's fears that she was experiencing stroke symptoms, an otherwise irreproachably caring physician rudely told him to tell her: "That's a lot of nonsense." The gentleman has told countless people about that one single miserable moment, and all too few people about the many magical ones.

That's why, in our attempts to be a go-beyond service business, The Williamsport Hospital & Medical Center stresses getting it right on each of the three dimensions of quality described in our quality rule 5 and on rewarding those who, in Ellen Goodman's words, "struggle to make one small difference after another" to avoid any bad surprises for the customer. And so, day in and day out, we convey the same message to our employees: Delivering go-beyond quality means multiplying and proliferating good surprises *and* eliminating, or at least drastically reducing, bad surprises.

QUALITY RULE 5: Keep Improving
the Three Things That Matter

The way we look at it, the name of the game is enthusiastic customers who feel good about all the important aspects of a service. CQI is the way one plays the game. In our view, the three critical dimensions that must be continually improved to delight customers are: the quality of the interactions between employees and customers (as mentioned we call this dimension C.A.R.E. for courtesy, attentiveness, responsiveness, and empathy), the customer friendliness of the service systems through which your employees render their services, TQM, and the ensured favorable technical outcome of the service (in the healthcare setting, we call this dimension MEDIMPROVE).

Customers we typically become regulars when all three dimension of a service go well. A hospital doesn't get a four-star rating if its medical outcomes are superior, the staff is considerate and caring, but access is difficult, waits are long, or services are not coordinated. Patients will not be repeat business if things go smoothly, the care is technically competent, but the staff is indifferent. And most assuredly, no one in the know will continue to get their services at any hospital if the service and the people are great, but the medical care is below par. To be successful, hospitals must score well on all three dimensions of quality. In baseball, three strikes and you're out. In a hospital, one strike and you're out.

At our hospital, we're really big on C.A.R.E. The C.A.R.E. dimension of quality has to do with tailor-made just-as-you-like-it personal services that accommodate individual preferences. The most important customer C.A.R.E. expectations occur during select key moments of truth in the cycle of service. As quality pioneer Tom Peters never tires of repeating in his talks: "No matter what your business is—if you treat your customers with ordinary, garden-variety courtesy, you'd have the lion's share of your market because you'd stand alone!" The TQM dimension of quality has to do with providing customer-friendly service delivery *systems* that ensure invariability, consistency, predictability, and dependability. The most important customer TQM expectations occur while customers are experiencing quality-critical processes. Last, the outcome or technical dimension of quality—what we've dubbed MEDIMPROVE in our hospital setting—has to do with a

11

favorable outcome and expert technique. At our hospital, we've identified the customer's most important MEDIMPROVE expectation to be what the Joint Commission on the Accreditation of Healthcare Organizations calls high-volume, high-cost, or problem-prone diagnoses and therapies. The three dimensions of quality and customers' most important expectations for each are detailed in the next chapter.

QUALITY RULE 6: If It Ain't Perfect, Make It Better

Peter Drucker has always been a favorite guru of our hospital's corporate staff. Years ago, he observed that organizations do only two things: marketing and innovation. By marketing, Drucker meant identifying and responding to customer needs. By innovation, he meant devising new ways to meet (we prefer to say exceed) those needs. Our view of what the hospital as a business does coincides with Drucker's.

That's why we always liked and still quote a sound-bite attributed to Masaki Imai, a popular author on quality in Japan. According to Imai, "Westerners often say: 'If it ain't broke, don't fix it. Easterners, by contrast, say: 'If it ain't perfect, make it better.'" The mind set expressed in the first saying plays itself out organizationally as crisis service management—fixing things after they've gone wrong. The outlook embodied in the second saying is that of a business in which things are less likely to go wrong because they are always getting better—the kind of business we dreamed of becoming.

A hospital that tries to be perfect on an aspect of service that is important to the customer but not really important to the volume of business generated is a rare find. An example is a hospital that is the only act around for certain services—for example, blood marrow or kidney transplants. Patients have to go there if they want to receive these services. The patients may be generally pleased with the services they receive there, but they are also displeased with the aloofness and coolness of the staff. From the hospital's business point of view, things aren't broken. But things certainly are not perfect. In many of these so-called centers of excellence, the introduction of the first dimension of quality—C.A.R.E.—would be a formidable task that runs against the grain of a deeply embedded culture of personal indifference. Give me the kindest, cleanest hospital with the best food in the country—if they're perfect in those aspects, I'll bet they're perfect in all aspects.

Several years ago, Mercedes Benz was working with a promotional agency on a new ad campaign for the glossy weeklies like *Time, Newsweek,* and *U.S. News and World Report.* At a meeting attended by representatives from every division of Mercedes, a presenter from the ad agency displayed a striking picture of a speeding sleek Mercedes sedan. The ad representative explained that her agency was considering the following test under the colorful picture of the car: "At seventy miles an hour, the only noise that can be heard in the soft, lush, plush, luxurious interior of a Mercedes Benz is the soft ticking of the dashboard clock." The woman had scarcely finished her last sentence before a Mercedes engineer chimed in: "We've got to do something about that damn clock!"

We realized that the pragmatist's reaction to this quintessential CQI mentality is that it is idealistic and ultimately doomed to disappointment and frustration. Herein lies the most stubborn obstacle to sustained quality efforts. Deep down within each of us resides a basic conservative belief that is hard to argue with: given the limitations of human nature, changes that bring about genuine improvement are almost always very difficult to bring about. Ever try to lose weight, control your temper, or stop smoking? Try to change an irritating habit in your mate? Try to get a military-style manager to become more collegial and participative? The disparity between the tremendous effort and time put into improving anything often seems way out of whack with the apparently puny successes achieved. Is CQI worth the effort?

Our way out of this dilemma was a strong belief in the principle of the fasces. The ancient Roman symbol of the fasces—a number of rods tied together by leather thongs around an axe—expressed the belief that the result of coordinated efforts exceeds the sum of each individual's contribution. A single rod could be easily broken. But, as one rod was added to another, there came a point at which they could no longer be broken. Small, seemingly insignificant single actions taken together can produce stupendous results. Two-plus-two can be made to equal five, or even six. The synergism of unified individual CQI efforts delivers remarkable service outcomes disproportionately more substantial than their originating service input. We know that the fasces is more than an evocative image because at The Williamsport Hospital & Medical Center, we've seen it come true.

Imagine for example what employees (notice I didn't say average employees) would think when they are challenged to acknowledge, smile at, and greet everyone they meet in the hospital—everyone, patients, family members, guests, physicians, vendors, people looking for a job—everyone. "So what's that going to do?" In a way, they are right. If only isolated individuals did that, the weight loss wouldn't be worth the diet. But if every employee did it day in and day out—the way they do at The Williamsport Hospital & Medical Center, within a year a hospital might be viewed as a friendly place. Heroes are individuals who do big things. Unsung heroes are individuals who do small worthy things well together always.

QUALITY RULE 7: Treat Your Employees Like Gold

If the deepest meaning of the Bible can best be summarized in the golden rule: "Love your neighbor as yourself," the rock-bed belief of our CQI efforts can best be summarized in these words addressed to our employees in one of our corporate objectives: "We promise to treat you the way we ask you to treat our patients."

We believe that the flip side of excellent customer relations is excellent employee relations. In service businesses, people make a distinctive contribution. A customer's perception of quality depends far more on employee excellence in a service industry than it does in a manufacturing plant. The conventional wisdom (85 percent to 90 percent of service problems occur because of faulty systems, not people) may not be as accurate in a service setting as it is in production settings. Over the long run, the way employees feel is the way customers will feel. The better your organizational climate assessments, the better your customer survey results.

I've heard Don Creamer say it a hundred times: "The reason we are a class act is very simple. When I spend time as chairman of the Hospital Association of Pennsylvania, I know our customers are being cared for by the corporate staff I chose myself, by a management staff that they put together and by an employee group—over 10 years diminished by more than 250 who didn't make the grade—who make you feel that you are a special someone when you give us the privilege of caring for you." Don was out yesterday. While he was gone, among other things, Jeannie Hill, our vice-president of nursing drove 10 miles to the home of a patient who indicated on her patient survey that she was displeased with her stay. We expect that patient to come back again. On that same day, four of our department heads, Bob Kane from the Emergency Services Department, Mark Grace from our Chaplaincy Services Department, Kim Peters from Nursing, and Mary Chancellor from Cancer Services headed up four different CQI groups. Throughout the house, on that same day, eight magic moments were reported. No doubt in my mind, literally hundreds of others occurred.

The president of Southwest Airlines underscored the absolute indispensability of top-flight employees in delivering go-beyond quality when he told *Aviation Week:* "Southwest has its customers—the passengers—and I have mine—the airline's employees. If the passengers aren't satisfied, they won't fly with us. If the employees aren't satisfied, they won't provide the service our customers require. Managers in our company are here to support the working troops, not vice versa." What applies to an airline applies to a hospital and to every other kind of service industry. The connection between employee enthusiasm and customer enthusiasm is so close, I have devoted an entire chapter to creating and maintaining a quality culture and ethic among service employees.

QUALITY RULE 8: Service Managers—Approve Them, Improve Them, Move Them, or Remove Them

The only way to treat employees like gold is to make sure each of them has an excellent manager. We tell our employees that, as part of their benefit package, they have a right to an excellent manager. Delivering on this promise is, by far, the most difficult part of our CQI work.

Everyone who completes the mandatory basic leadership course at The Williamsport Hospital & Medical Center knows that managers are responsible for results. Specifically, managers are expected to ensure that their customers actually receive—and perceive they receive—personally attentive (C.A.R.E.), hassle-free (TQM), and medically efficacious (MEDIMPROVE) healthcare services. They are held accountable for the objective outcomes our customers receive and for the subjective outcomes our customers experience.

You can't hold employees to the highest standards of quality if you tolerate mediocre, not to mention inferior, service managers. In the words of my boss, Don Creamer: "You can't ask eagles to soar if they're led by a turkey." C.A.R.E. starts with managerial C.A.R.E. for employees, not employee C.A.R.E. for customers. TQM starts with the *M,* not the *TQ.* And MEDIMPROVE starts with managerial standards of excellence. Quality is like a game of pool and the manager is the cue stick.

The business of our hospital *is* quality and the existing hierarchically ordered managerial team *is* the service quality leadership. If an executive, a manager, or a supervisor will not or cannot serve as a quality team leader, he is in the wrong job. The task here is approve them, improve them, move them, or remove them:

- Step 1—approve them. Make an explicit decision that they can motivate members of their team to consistently deliver go-beyond quality.
- Step 2—improve them. Train them, coach them, and assist them.
- Step 3—If, after every effort is made, managers still can't effectively play their required quality leadership role, try to match their interest and skills to another job.
- Step 4—remove them. If a transfer cannot be effected, we reluctantly but unfailingly terminate unsuccessful service managers. We consider a willingness to be hard regarding our corporate value as the litmus test of the depth of our commitment to quality.

Managing favorable subjective outcomes is not a delegatable managerial responsibility. It *is* a manager's job. Companies that refuse to transform or replace ineffective service team leaders aren't really serious about CQI. They fail the quality litmus test. In these competitive times, organizations that are not ready to deal with their managerial turkeys ought to get ready for "the turkey shoot."

QUALITY RULE 9: CQI + CPI = CVI

I must confess . . . I'm not prone to take much of what economists have to say very seriously, but I do think economists are onto something important when they talk about something they call factor price equalization. In *Head to Head* (William Morrow, 1992), Lester Thurow from MIT explains this scary-sounding concept quite simply: "Economic activity won't be in any geographic location unless that location is the least cost location for producing that particular product. The capitalist who is willing to work for the lowest rate of return in the world sets the maximum return for everybody else."

The real players in the service quality arena may not know the academic language, but they sure know that quality alone is not enough. For a business to succeed, quality needs to be married to price to give birth to value. Consequently, first-rate companies are obsessed with continuous value improvement (CVI)—that is, quality at competitive prices, and not just with continuous quality improvement (CQI).

A fixation on quality at class-act companies is linked to a hard-nosed, even wiley, realism about price reminiscent of this story: A reporter asked a 100-year-old man about the secret of his long life. The old man hesitated and then answered calculatingly: "I'm not sure yet. I'm still negotiating with a cereal company and a company that sells exercise equipment."

In healthcare, unless we dramatically improve on delivering value for the dollar, we're likely to break the federal treasury and render our business customers internationally noncompetitive. Our gross domestic product is $6 trillion a year. We spend about $1 trillion of it on healthcare. In 1992, we spend about $3,400 a year per person on healthcare. Japan spent $785. If current trends continue, we will have to spend $47,000 a year per person by the year 2030. No way customers will allow that to happen! Healthcare customers, especially payors like the government, employers, and individuals expect value—not just quality at any cost. So do the purchasers of every other service I can think of. Companies that successfully practice CVI will be the ones that get and keep their business—that is, Continuous Quality Improvement plus continuous price improvement.

QUALITY RULE 10: What Counts Is Execution, Not Elocution

"Easier said than done." "Talk is cheap." "Walk the talk." The concept is far from new. As Portia says to Nerissa in *The Merchant of Venice:* "If to do were as easy as it is to know what it were good to do, chapels would be churches and poor men's cottages, princes' palaces." In 1984, Harold Geeneen, Chairman of ITT said it anew for our times: "It is an immutable law of business that words are words, explanations are explanations, promises are promises—but only performance is reality." Whatever the language, especially with quality, execution, not elocution, is what matters.

In our attempts to translate the rhetoric of quality into the daily habitual practice of quality, we have tried to develop two essential dispositions in all of our employees: a can-do attitude and a want-to attitude.

Quality leaders tend to underestimate the capability and potential of their employees. Most employee groups can do a bang-up job by their customers if their managers set and support the implementation of high standards of service. People tend to become what you tell them they are. I, for one, would match the employees at our hospital with employees anywhere. I've told our people that a million times. After a visit from a CEO and his new vice-president for human resources from another hospital, the vice-president called me and said: "My boss told me that my new job could be summed up in one sentence, 'I want you to make our employees like their employees.' " I asked him what he meant. He said our hospital was the friendliest one he had ever been in. "It's a lot more than this, Tim," he said, "but everyone, I mean everyone here always greets you—always. How in the world do you folks make that happen?"

"The fault, dear Brutus, is not in our stars but in ourselves that we are underlings," Cassius says in *Julius Caesar.* The reason within ourselves for our failure to achieve our quality potential is that we set service goals that do not challenge our people. Being able to do something doesn't mean you will do it. You've got to want to before you truly can. Getting people to want to (not finding people who can) is the real challenge. In their most unguarded thoughts, employees ask: "How am I doing? Where am I going? And what's in it for me?" Sustained motivation of employees toward a quality service ideal is possible only when employees believe there is an alignment between their own personal and professional aspirations and a business's quality ideals.

CQI is first and foremost a cultural and motivational transformation—and only secondarily a scientific methodology using statistical tools to continually improve service systems. The introduction of TQM tools to improve service systems before the permeation of a quality belief system is like planting seeds in clay without fertilizing and preparing the soil.

QUALITY RULE 11: Install a Quality Model That Fits

Making cars and providing financial services. Manufacturing rods for nuclear plants and running a hotel. Producing soda cans and treating patients. It still perplexes me to see so many service-sector businesses using quality models originating in the process-fixated, zero-defect environments of manufacturing plants as their principal paradigm.

Until recently, in manufacturing settings, the single-minded goal of CQI used to be to reduce variability in all processes. That is why systems were so important there and the general rule was to allow relatively low worker discretion—usually only when the system created an error. Today, even on the plant floor, the worker's special quality role is being recognized. In service settings, one goal of CQI is TQM: the reduction of variability in selected processes (e.g., medical procedures or regimens with strictly prescribed standards—such as administering an intravenous treatment). But another goal of CQI in places like a hospital is custom-tailoring services to meet special needs—making choices about variability (e.g., when and how to get an objecting patient to allow the insertion of an intravenous needle). That's why people are important and why we empower people by encouraging high worker discretion when circumstances call for it.

No two patients are alike. No two customers are alike. No two moments of truth are alike. The delivery of a service and the reception of a service are simultaneous. There is no time lapse between the two to inspect for quality as there is between the manufacture and use of a product. No one can make a well-delivered service unsatisfactory, and no one can transform a poorly delivered service into a good one. Either your employees are your inspectors or you don't have inspectors. In a hospital, the customers' perception of service quality depends far more on employee excellence than in manufacturing industries.

The state-of-the-art in service excellence provides an overall conceptualization of quality initiatives that pay due regard to the distinctive contribution of people to the service experience and the opportunity to adopt and adapt selected tools from the process-minded manufacturing setting in improving service delivery systems.

CQI cannot happen without people. CQI cannot last without institutionalization. Translating the high-sounding principles outlined in this chapter requires the institutional integration of practices and programs that support the three dimensions of quality: C.A.R.E., TQM, and MEDIMPROVE. At our hospital, for example, C.A.R.E. is guaranteed eternal life by our C.A.R.E. award program. TQM and MED-IMPROVE have an assured perpetual existence through our cycle of service teams, our departmental CQI teams, our chairman's award program, and our CQI SWAT teams. In addition, MEDIMPROVE is sure to last because all of the activities of every patient care committee are guided and coordinated by the hospital's MEDIMPROVE CQI steering committee.

QUALITY RULE 12: High-Quality Service Must Be Preceded and Supported by High-Quality Strategic Planning

One Sunday afternoon, the Brown's quarterback, Brian Sipe, was having a particularly bad day. As Brian trudged off the field after his fifth interception, his coach Sam Rutigliano grabbed him by the arm and demanded in exasperation, "Brian, why do you keep throwing the ball to the guys on the other team?" Brain retorted, "Because they're the only ones open!"

All of the well-intentioned, talented people in the world can't make up for poor strategic planning. Sure there were other problems, but when American steel executives decided to stick with outmoded blast furnaces instead of installing the open hearth furnaces the Japanese and Europeans were installing in the early 1950s, the industry set the competitive time-bomb that virtually decimated the industry in the next two decades. When U.S. auto manufacturers decided in the late 1970s that Americans wouldn't drive compact cars, they began the trend that has culminated in a more than 35% Japanese share of this country's automobile market. When inventors failed to develop marketing strategies, the Japanese landed up selling almost all of the quartz watches invented in Switzerland, the compact discs invented in the Netherlands, and the videotape recorders invented in the United States.

High-quality strategic planning provides the opportunity to deliver high-quality services the way a well-conceived offensive game plan gives a quarterback the opportunity to throw a completion to an open receiver. Doing the right thing gives you the chance to do things the right way. In the film *Gettysburg,* John Buford especially and officers from the North and the South made much about the fighting on good or high ground—that is, on elevated terrain. Soldiers on both sides of that fateful three-day battle were their states' best. But the day was won by the North when General Lee decided to attack the good ground staked out by General Meade.

In healthcare, strategic planning works from the right kind of mission, value, and vision statements through an analysis of local, regional, and national trends that reveal market opportunities and threats to detailed long- and short-term goals, objectives, and a detailed strategy about the institution's market position and niches, managed care approach, product lines, collaborative and employment relations with physicians, other healthcare institutions, providers and referral sources, human resources mix, allocation and location, competitive posture, and facility master plan. Even the best soldiers in the best of armies may fail if the enemy has the advantage of good ground. So, too, with top-of-the-line employees; they need a quality strategic plan if they are to have a chance to deliver go-beyond service.

Here's an example of what I mean. You are Hospital A. You are definitely the hi-touch hospital. Your competitor, Hospital B, is unquestionably the hi-tech place. You work hard to transform yourself into a hi-tech place not measurably distinguishable from your competitor. Your care-givers outservice your competitors daily. However, you have not successfully established the managed care relationships needed with physicians and a with a competitive and effectively marketed healthcare plan. Overall, you have the better service. But you don't have the high ground. Under these conditions, your employees may perform marvelously. But institutionally, you may not prevail.

In the remainder of this book, I will describe how The Williamsport Hospital & Medical Center has applied these 12 quality rules in its efforts to make repeat business of each and every one of its customers.

Chapter 2 covers the organizational foundations we established to get our CQI effort organized and started. Chapter 3 describes how we developed and communicated our quality expectations. In chapter 4, we explain the ways we train all our employees to deliver go-beyond quality service daily in the three dimensions of quality. Chapter 5 presents the mechanisms through which we foster individual and team efforts in CQI. In chapter 6, we provide a detailed description of the means we use to motivate our managers and our employees to sustain our quality initiatives. Chapter 7 makes the case for the vital link we think exists between human resources and CQI. In the concluding chapters, chapter 8 and 9, we describe the quality destinations we have reached, the new quality routes we have yet to travel, and the obstacles and opportunities that lie ahead. In chapters 2 through 8, I provide tools we've used to promote the quality activities discussed in these chapters.

2

The Organizational and Managerial Foundations of Quality

"Quality initiatives are wasted efforts unless
the people who have to implement them believe in the
people leading the effort."

—James M. Kouzes and Barry Z. Posner

Stephen Covey and Keith Gulledge argue that the first responsibility of leadership is to establish True North or the identity of an institution: the mission and vision of the enterprise, including the principles and values upon which to base their fulfillment. Almost 10 years ago, The Williamsport Hospital & Medical Center established its True North:

> "To deliver go-beyond Quality and value that surpass customer expectations for personal service, user-friendly service systems, and favorable healthcare outcomes and processes through a three-pronged continuous quality improvement business strategy: C.A.R.E., TQM, and MEDIMPROVE."

Before we actually took off on our CQI mission, everyone within the hospital had to be prepared for the quality journey. By that time, I had adapted a program I had used in my previous job at the Frankford Hospital in Philadelphia.

Getting the Quality Word Out to Everyone

The loud buzzing tailed off to complete silence as I entered the hospital's mini-amphitheater. It was September 1984, my second month at the hospital. I had already given the two session seven-hour program introducing our quality C.A.R.E. program (*C*ourtesy, *A*ttentiveness, *R*esponsiveness, and *E*mpathy) to members of the hospital's trustees and management staff. The participants before me were the first employees and volunteers to attend the quality kick-off sessions I would be giving over the next six months. (see Resource 2-1).

"Well," I began, "You've all read about C.A.R.E. recently in our hospital's newsletter. What do you think?" "Yes," I said to a gentleman from maintenance in the back row. "I think it's a crock," he responded. "Oookay," I sputtered as I thought, There's only one way to go from here—and that's up.

"How about the rest of you?" I went on, feigning nonchalance that belied my fear I might not emerge from the session in one piece. "What's your gimmick going to be five years from now?" an otherwise

---

Resource 2-1. Content for the Kick-Off Sessions on Quality C.A.R.E.

The opening sessions on quality C.A.R.E. are designed so that participants:

- Understand and are committed to a customer centered work ethic ("Remember the Shoe").
- Are resolved to improve their own personal behavior and involvement in providing quality care ("Remember *Your Own* Cookie Bag").
- Dedicate themselves to go-beyond quality ("Make Our Hospital more like heaven than hell").
- Promise to emulate four key behaviors that embody C.A.R.E.
- Are familiarized with the 25 C.A.R.E. behaviors as specific expectations for their daily performance.

friendly looking woman asked. The rest of the questions and comments from the floor were in the same vein. This was not going to be a quick fix, I remember thinking, and we're going to have to stick to and build upon what we begin with. There would have to be continuity in our continuous quality objectives, approach, and communications. Otherwise, folks would justifiably think: This is the flavor of the month. What'll it be next year?

The corporate staff imagined quality training to be an unending song not an endless string or programs *du jour.* The kick-off sessions constituted the chorus containing themes that were to be incessantly repeated throughout all ensuing training. They viewed all of the other subsequent training as new verses to the same song. The seven themes in the kick-off chorus were:

An inspiring, unifying vision and belief system: Treat our customers like gold

We stand for and work to create patients and customers so enthused about our C.A.R.E.ing style, our hassle-free delivery systems and healthcare outcomes that they and their families become our loyal lifetime clientele whose word-of-mouth advertising makes promotion superfluous. We are all about ensuring objectively-based, favorably perceived customer service experiences that prompt our customers to say, "Wow!"

A personal commitment to demonstrate C.A.R.E. (courtesy, attentiveness, responsiveness, and empathy) metanoia service

Peter Senge calls the drastic personal change required as a prerequisite to quality service metanoia—a Biblical term meaning conversion or radical change in behavior. Everyone has got to come away from the kick-off training believing that they *really* count. The voluntary gift of every individual to do his or her best by the customer is indispensable to achieving a hospital's quality ideal. Our way of getting this idea across to our people is the story behind the friendly piece of advice: "Remember Your Own Cookie Bag." (See Resource 2-A in the Appendix for this story and those referred to here. It's The Williamsport

Hospital and Medical Center culture to use stories to communicate important themes in a memorable and fun way.)

A personal promise to bend over backward to render go-beyond quality

This is accomplished by being the customer's servant. Meeting customers' basic needs, expectations, and desires won't do. Customer satisfaction is for organizations who are happy to place or show. Winners seek to surprise the customer—to transform key moments of truth into magic moments—by doing the unanticipated. Winners create enthusiastic customers, not satisfied ones. We convey this ideal through a provocative description of heaven and hell.

An understanding that quality is a together thing

Individual commitment and effort are indispensable for quality to happen, but they are not sufficient. Success comes only through the synergism of joint, collaborative, teamwork—people working together within and across departments. Individuals must submerge purely individualistic goals for commonly shared customer-focused goals. As our president and CEO, Don Creamer tells our employees: "Teamwork makes quality possible. Teamwork is the ability to work together toward a common vision—to consider organizational objectives and patient expectations over individual accomplishments and self-interest. It is what allows ordinary people, working together, to achieve extraordinary results." We like to remind our people of the team dimension of quality by constantly invoking "The Refrigerator" story (see page 238) and "The Principle of the Fasces" (see page 13).

A belief that employees, too, will benefit from a joint effort at making quality a daily occurrence

An employee may not articulate it in such straightforward language, but every employee thinks: How am I doing? Where am I going, and what's in it for me? Is quality C.A.R.E. something I've got to do for others, period—or will it also be extended to me? Is there any alignment between my personal and professional aspirations and the hospital's quality goals? To these questions, the hospital said: "We promise to treat you the way we ask you to treat our patients—with C.A.R.E."

A resolve to transform undesirable feelings into desirable ones through positive behaviors and to project caring through non-verbal communication

People usually act the way they feel, and actions are often dictated by emotions. Psychologists tell us we can affect the way we feel by the way we act. We challenge our employees to reverse the feelings/actions connection and to refuse to have their behaviors dictated by their feelings.

Other psychologists, like Albert Mehrabian, tell us that much of what we convey to others is communicated nonverbally and that the most important attitudes we project are communicated in that way. Specifically, through nonverbal communication, we convey:

- the degree to which we like or dislike others.
- the degree to which we consider ourselves to be superior to, inferior to, or on a par with others.
- the degree to which we are interested in other people's problems and concerns—the degree to which we care.

We teach our employees to communicate the following attitudes nonverbally to everyone they encounter: "I like you." "I'm just like you." "I care about you."

Personal changes immediately affecting behaviors that are cues to quality

What are these behaviors? First, acknowledge, smile and greet *everyone* you pass. Imagine it: 1,500 employees times, for example, 20 people, times 240 days a year. That's more than 7 million encounters a year for starters. *Atmospheres are created by behaviors—not by accident!* Second, pepper your language with the magic phrases: please, thank you, you're welcome, and I'm sorry. Use people's names. Third, directions: Every lost person is an opportunity for a magic moment. Look for them! Take them where they need to go if you can. Hook them up with someone else if you can't. Give clear, helpful directions as a minimum. And fourth, the 25 C.A.R.E. behaviors.

The strategy for the kick-off session was to be heavy on the what and the why of quality and on the how of customer-directed personal behaviors. The idea was to pick the easy fruit from the low branches: employee and volunteer interpersonal behaviors directed at patients, families, and guests—behaviors that happen to coincide with high-priority customer expectations and aspects of service that customers are capable of evaluating and typically do evaluate.

Employees willing to change their own personal behavior on behalf of the patient, the corporate staff reasoned, would later be willing to change service systems and healthcare protocols on their behalf as well.

THE BOARD'S JOB:
Seeing to It That Quality Is a Corporate Mandate

About the only thing a board can do to make sure a hospital reaches its full quality potential and gain the resulting customer satisfaction and financial and clinical outcomes is to hire someone who is willing and able to undertake the long and painstaking task of building a management team that will help create the culture from which go-beyond quality springs.

In April 1984, the board of managers at The Williamsport Hospital & Medical Center hired such a person as its president and CEO, Donald R. Creamer. Don lead the board to define the hospital's:

- Mission as a commitment to quality and to the processes by which quality is managed.
- Value as a promise to treat employees and customers like gold.
- Goals to provide customers with service experiences that lead to objective customer enthusiasm.
- Business strategy as synonymous with continuous quality improvement.
- Service focus as customer value priorities—that is, key moments of truth in the cycle of service for all interpersonal interactions, quality-critical processes in service delivery systems and high-

cost, high-volume, problem-prone diagnosis for medical outcomes and processes.

- Employees unified in pursuit of CQI as the key link between the organization's focus on high-priority customer needs and the organization's response of go-beyond value.

In a word, Don lead the board to articulate and promulgate quality as a corporate mandate.

Don then structured all of his individual and committee contacts with the board in ways that would allow board members to understand, provide input, and evaluate the hospital's ongoing efforts to make this corporate mandate a reality through institutionally integrated practices that support each of the three dimensions of go-beyond Quality:

- personal service (C.A.R.E.),
- customer friendly service systems (TQM or reengineering), and
- favorable health outcomes (MEDIMPROVE).

Don and other members of the corporate staff spend at least five hours explaining and discussing quality as the hospital's business strategy with every newly appointed member of the hospital's Board of Managers. The board and all of its committees typically conduct their business as CQI monitors of the hospital's efforts to maintain superlative services. The principal focus of the hospital's two-and-a-half-day joint board/corporate staff retreat is always on *value*—that is, the quality and cost efficiency of the hospital's services and operations. The chairman of the board personally and publicly bestows the most prestigious individual award for quality (C.A.R.E. Employee of the Year Award) and the most highly sought group award for quality (The Chairman's Award for CQI Improvement of the Year). Through practices such as these, Don helps the board members view themselves as having ultimate fiduciary responsibility for interpersonal, system, and medical quality—the very definition of the hospital's business. Led by Dick DeWald, Dean Fisher, Jim Kauffman, Jim Wirt, Ron DeFeo, and Jim Lamade, with competent guidance by physicians like Bill Beltz, M.D., Timothy Pagana, M.D., Marcia Finn, M.D., and William Judson, M.D., The Williamsport Hospital & Medical Center's Board of Managers serve as admirable stewards of the hospital's quality ideals.

SENIOR MANAGEMENT'S JOB:
Making Quality Happen Hospitalwide

In a recent article, "Employee Commitment: Managing Quality, Culture & the Bottom Line," in *Dialogue* (Summer 1993), in an Epic Care Health Group study, Joe Philip concluded that employees with high levels of commitment to the company believe:

- Hospital management is interested in their welfare.
- Hospital management is committed to providing quality patient care.
- The hospital lives up to its guiding principles.
- Communications about what is going on in the hospital are effective.

During his first two years, Don Creamer rebuilt his corporate team. He designated the corporate staff as the hospital's quality council. As the hospital's quality council, corporate staff was from the beginning responsible for directing and coordinating all of the CQI efforts hospitalwide. With staff work done by a steering committee, the MEDIMPROVE committee (on which seven corporate staff members serve), the corporate quality council fulfills its role by:

- Participating in an annual two-day corporate/board planning advance (what others often call retreats), which initiates the planning cycle, plans service gap closure, and sets directions for implementing the hospital's mission statement, corporate value statement, corporate goals and objectives, and long-range plan.
- Communicating the annual corporate strategic plan elements and the update of the long-range plan to staff and operations departments for their use in planning.
- Overseeing the annual update of the quality service plan, which consists of the individual service plans of every staff and operations department of the hospital.
- Commissioning and monitoring the progress of self-managing CQI teams with interdepartmental representation and a cross-organizational cycle of service focus.

- Evaluating and approving the budget requests of the CQI teams.
- Serving as the judging panel for the hospital's annual quality service awards competition (i.e., The Chairman's Quality Award).

Corporate staff members are held directly responsible for the quality of the services provided to customers and for the morale and motivation of employees in the departments reporting to them. They receive ongoing feedback and an extensive formal annual evaluation from the hospital's president and CEO on their effectiveness as members of the quality council and on their success in achieving the hospital's quality goals in the departments that report to them (see Resource 2-B). Their annual merit increases are based largely on their participation in and success at putting into practice the hospital's quality standards.

Hospital corporate officers, managers, and supervisors are enlisted to become models of quality care behavior by devoting appreciable portions of their scheduled time to the quality care effort, by acting as service managers, rather than aloof office managers, and by embodying the C.A.R.E. behaviors. "The most dangerous place from which to view the world," we often say, "is from behind a desk." Employees do what we do, not what we say.

Imitative learning was deemed from the start of our program to be the principal vehicle in any sustained quality care effort. Consequently, in words describing the new management style at the big three car makers, *modesty, humor* (especially of the self-deprecating variety), *open discussion, candor,* and *team play* are in. *Pomp, protocol, pretension,* and *paperwork* are out.

THE DEPARTMENT HEAD'S JOB:
Making Quality Happen Within and Among Departments

A fairly strident and pervasive theme throughout the management literature of the 1980s was that mid-level managers are superfluous. If you have got to cut, that's were you do it.

From all of our previous experience, members of the corporate staff did not believe that this newly discovered managerial dogma was applicable in our hospital setting, whatever worth it might have in other environments. As a matter of fact, we thought the opposite was

31

true: regardless of how talented a corporate staff member was, departmental service quality and employee morale never reached their full potential unless a department was led by a highly competent department head.

One of our clinical departments was run by a department head with clinical credentials, experience, and accomplishments seldom seen in others in his field. He is an invaluable—I would say irreplaceable talent—but he was playing the wrong position. All of his supervisors were clinically competent, but organizationally divisive. A typical remark: "I think it's stupid, but this is what *they* want *us* to do." The vice-president in charge spent an inordinate amount of time working directly with this department, all to no avail. Inpatient and outpatient volumes went to all-time lows. The department had the lowest climate assessment ratings in the entire hospital.

We made one of our best managers the new department head. We made the previous department head our clinical director—he is now a star! One of our supervisors got religion and is now a model team leader in this department. Three supervisors have moved on as they say, "to explore other business opportunities." The rest is history. Dramatically improved patient outcomes against outcomes in a national data base. Record volumes. The best climate assessment ratings of any large department in the hospital. No question about it in our minds: the key to intra-departmental service excellence and interdepartmental service coordination is the presence of highly competent interpersonally skilled department heads.

Based on this view of the department head's role and importance, in 1984, the hospital's corporate staff began an annual process that came to be called "approve them, improve them, move them, or remove them." Before vice-presidents give individual department heads their annual measurable performance evaluations, the entire corporate staff offers input from their perspective on the technical competence, managerial effectiveness, interpersonal behavior, and departmental service quality of each department head. After extensive discussions about each department head, the corporate staff annually places them into one of three scientifically based and empirically supported categories: the good, the bad, and the ugly. Individual corporate staff members are assigned the responsibility of moving those in the bad or ugly categories over to the good column by:

Improving them

Corporate Staff members are asked to give these departments heads advice and coaching on how to improve, help to improve, time to improve, and feedback on progress (see Resource 2-2).

Just this past year, for example, one of our vice-presidents and two human resources staff members worked the entire year with a technically competent, personably affable department head with less than adequate communication systems and skills. The department head still has a way to go, but the year brought tremendous progress. With continued support, we are optimistic that we will soon be dealing with a fresh success story.

Moving them

If reasonable efforts at improving are not successful, corporate staff members are asked to consider the possibility of moving department heads to positions that more closely match their talents, abilities, and interests—if such positions are open.

There are about six people at The Williamsport Hospital & Medical Center who informally serve as the principal catalysts in activating our managers to make quality their job and to do a quality job. One of these indispensable quality leaders moved from a position that was not an ideal match for his skills to a job that capitalizes on his considerable strengths. He's happy. And believe me, as we consider his tremendous contributions, we are too.

Removing them

Should efforts at improving fail and opportunities for moving are not available, corporate staff members are asked to work on outplacing department heads who cannot meet their responsibilities to deliver quality service within their departments.

As chief operating officer and vice-president for clinical services respectively, Steve Johnson and Jeannie Hill have led the corporate staff in creatively and successfully working with the largest number of managers needing support because of serious performance gaps. For example, one of her managers had serious problems organizing herself and her

---

Resource 2-2.   Guidelines for Developing Managers in Need of Improvement

As managers of managers, corporate staff officers need to do more than point out performance deficiencies and inadequacies. They need to serve as coaches and mentors in response to the basic rights managers, like other employees, enjoy at The Williamsport Hospital & Medical Center:

1. *Managers have a right to notice and feedback.* As Ken Blanchard has often remarked: The most widespread form of management style in America is "leave-alone-zap"—characterized by a lack of timely feedback and, once things deteriorate to a level of unacceptability, drastic intervention like termination. Employees need feedback as soon as patterns of undesirable performance are noticed.

2. *Managers have the right to know what standards are expected.* In setting out clear performance expectations, we ask managers to follow the model for defining expectations set out in the *One-Minute Manager:* expectations should be delineated as SMART goals:
    * *S*pecific.
    * *M*easurable.
    * *A*greed upon.
    * *R*easonable
    * *T*rackable.

3. *Managers have a right to a chance to improve.* The first kind of organizational intervention ought to be a genuine effort to improve performance. The last reluctant resort is to remove the person.

4. *Managers have a right to help to improve.* Many floundering managers can't get back on the right track by themselves. Never during their careers are struggling managers more in need of their own manager's support and guidance.

5. *Managers have a right to have sufficient time to carry out the prescribed improvements.*

staff. Jeannie ensured that she was tutored in project and time management. Another manager was perceived as uncaring by her staff. Jeannie personally taught her relational behaviors that effective managers practice with their associates and continued to give her feedback on her progress.

Over the past 10 years we have been gratified to find that many of our department heads could be brought up to acceptable levels of performance through management development and training. Some others—typically shortstops playing first base—have had the opportunity to switch over to positions for which they are better equipped and disposed to fill. Some others were never able to live up to their responsibilities as service managers and team builders and were consequently separated from employment at the hospital. For example, we have transferred misplaced managers into staff positions and dismissed those whose interpersonal relations with their staff did not meet our standards even after attempts at improvement.

As a result of the approve them, move them, improve them, or remove them process, only 6 members of the combined corporate and department head staff are now in the positions they held 10 years ago. Virtually all of the combined corporate and department head staff are still in the positions they were in seven years ago. However Draconian this process may seem, total quality cannot be held up as an ideal if less than total quality managers are tolerated over long periods of time. To repeat: TQM in our mind begins with the *M* not with the *TQ*. You cannot ask eagles to sore if they are lead by a turkey.

GETTING TO KNOW THE CUSTOMER:
Customer Research Tools

Corporate staff held four unshakable beliefs about being a market- or customer-driven organization:

- The single most important measure of service quality is the quality of service perceived by the customer compared to one's competitor.
- Market research must provide detailed information on customer needs—not just on customer satisfaction—to plan future CQI initiatives.

- The key differentiating factor between companies whose quality efforts have succeeded and those that have not is that successful businesses remain fixed primarily on customer outcomes as an end and process improvement as a means.
- Quality organizations differentiate the very most important and urgent customer needs from among other merely important customer needs and concentrate their resources on these highest priority expectations.

As vice-president for marketing, Bill McClain has been the architect of bringing our customers into the heart of the business's service quality decision-making process through his leadership in implementing ongoing efforts to ascertain the customer's needs and expectations. To maintain our hospital as an outside-in kind of business, we regularly use a wide range of research tools (see Resource 2-3). They are all designed to keep us moving away from "Here's what we have, let's promote it," to "Here's what the people we serve have told us they need, let's meet those needs."

DEFINING THE CQI INITIATIVE:
Approach and Dimensions

As we said in chapter 1, customers typically evaluate services first in this way: "Was I treated well?" In our language, "Did I receive *C*ourtesy, *A*ttentiveness, *R*esponsiveness, and *E*mpathy?" "Was I treated like a special someone?" "Did they try to do things the way I like them?" "Did they care?" There is an interpersonal dimension to quality.

Second, they ask: "Did things run smoothly?" In our language, "Did customers experience customer-friendly service systems?" "Did things go well at critical moments during the entire cycle of service?" There is a system dimension to quality service.

Third, "Did they help me solve my medical problem or help me avoid having a medical problem?" "Did I get well or stay well?" "Did they use up-to-date technology and procedures?" There is obviously a medical or healthcare dimension to quality service in a hospital setting.

Our go-beyond practices to support the interpersonal quality is called C.A.R.E. Practices to support the system dimension of service

---

Resource 2-3. Market Research Tools

For C.A.R.E. and TQM (customer relations and service systems quality processes):

- Customer satisfaction monitoring systems:
    —Inpatient Surveys
    —Outpatient Surveys
    —Hospitality Inn Surveys
    —Physician Surveys—General and service specific
    —Physician Office Staff Surveys
    —Physician Office Practice Patient Surveys
- Employee Climate Assessments.
- Market research and needs assessment studies—Identify needs, expectations, problems and preferences of specific market segments (e.g., women, seniors).
- Departmental and cross-organizational quality audits—These also address medical quality issues.
- Focus group studies.
- Management engineering studies of operational processes.
- Community advisory boards—These function as ongoing focus groups to address customer issues of specific market segments such as women, seniors, and business and industry.
- Competitor intelligence surveys—To identify hospital shortcomings and service gaps as perceived by patients who select other institutions.
- Community leadership breakfasts—To assess community leaders' (business, government, and civic) perceptions of the hospital and its services.
- Physician breakfast program.

For MEDIMPROVE (clinical/medical quality processes):

- Medisgroups—A national data base system for comparing clinical outcomes.
- VHA/PA Clinical Benchmarking Studies.
- Tumor registry.

Resource 2-3. Market Research Tools *(continued)*

**For MEDIMPROVE
(clinical/medical quality processes):**

- ORSOS—A system for evaluating operating room procedures in terms of staffing, resources, and costs.
- Functional Improvement Measurement System (FIMS)—A national comparative data base that permits The Williamsport Hospital & Medical Center to compare its inpatient rehabilitation results to those of other centers regionally and nationally.

---

quality are called TQM/Reengineering. Efforts to support the medical outcome and process dimension of quality are called MED-IMPROVE.

We use the following criteria to evaluate the C.A.R.E. dimension of our service delivery:

- *Reliability*—Was the service provided correctly and dependably the first time?
- *Tangibles*—Did they look good? Were the appearance, the facilities, the equipment, and verbal and nonverbal communication of the personnel indicative of a professional and quality service?
- *Responsiveness*—Were the staff members willing to go out of their way to help customers and provide prompt service?
- *Reassurance*—Did the staff project themselves as trustworthy, believable, and honest?
- *Empathy*—Did the staff provide the kind of caring and individualized attention they would like to have received themselves?

The criteria we use to evaluate the system and medical outcomes dimensions of our quality are derived from the quality cube published by the Joint Commission on the Accreditation of Healthcare Organizations:

- *Efficacy*—Did the intervention accomplish the desired result?
- *Appropriateness*—Was the intervention the best suited to the patient's clinical needs, given our current state of knowledge?

- *Availability*—Was the patient able to secure the needed service when he or she needed it?
- *Timeliness*—Was the required intervention provided when it was needed and when it was most beneficial to the patient?
- *Correctiveness*—Was the intervention provided done properly so that the desired outcome could be achieved?
- *Continuity*—Were the services coordinated over time among all the practitioners involved?
- *Safety*—Was the risk of the intervention reduced to acceptable levels for both the patient and the practitioners?
- *Efficiency*—Was there a commensurate relationship between the outcomes and the resources used to provide patient care?

We have also recently adopted the Joint Commission on the Accreditation of Healthcare Organization's 1994 manual to guide us in the organization or our quality efforts in all three dimensions of quality: C.A.R.E., TQM, and MEDIMPROVE:

- Improvement of organizational performance.
- Surveillance, prevention, and control of infections.
- Management of the environment of care.
- Management of human resources.
- Management of information.
- Leadership.
- Coordination of care.
- Education of patients and family.
- Operative and other invasive procedures.
- Treatment of patients.
- Nutritional care.
- Entry to setting or service.
- Assessment of patients.
- Health promotion and disease prevention.
- Rights of patients and organizational ethics.

We are particularly attracted to this functional catalog because it forces individual departments to view their services as multidisciplinary and interdepartmental. For example, the management of the environment of C.A.R.E. requires us to do more than exceed the aesthetic expectations of our customers. Our customers also have specialized medical, psychological, and even spiritual requirements. Therefore, for example, the applicable criteria for environmental CQI efforts require the inclusion of not only environmental services but also of staff like patient care givers, psychologists, infection control specialists, chaplaincy, risk management and safety and security. The remainder of this book provides examples of programs, practices, and tools that we have made part of the hospital's everyday life to ensure customer enthusiasm by exceeding the performance criteria for each of the dimensions of quality previously described.

TOTALLY MANAGING THE TWO RELATIONSHIPS THAT COUNT: Employees/Customers and Managers/Employees

The games of golf and table pool have the same objective: to get a ball into a hole. In golf, the player makes contact with only one ball and drives the ball directly toward the pin. In pool, the player contacts one ball directly and another indirectly. The player has to use the cue ball to hit the target ball. Managing quality is more like playing pool than it is like playing golf.

The cue ball is the employee; the target is the customer. The only way to get to the customer is through the employee. Employees transform moments of truth into magic moments for the customer. Employees create systems and processes that leave customers hassle-free. Employees are ultimately accountable for using the very best clinical pathways and procedures to achieve positive healthcare outcomes.

The hospital promises employees that they have a right to a good manager as part of their benefit package. Regular management development and training are offered to keep the caliber of managerial performance high. Managers are regularly evaluated on their relationships with their employees. Employees are given an annual opportunity to evaluate all levels of management, working conditions, and the quality of our customer services.

Employees are encouraged to submit questions, concerns, and suggestions to senior management and are guaranteed a corporate officer's response within five working days.

In just the past month, I have personally responded to the following kinds of impact statements:

- "I don't get paid enough. Check it out."
- "Some employees take patient parking places. Help."
- "Why can't I give Penelope my sick time? She's out."
- "If we're trying to save money, why do you have a picnic after the last management development program?"

Employees have easy access to all levels of management. The hospital fosters employee appreciation and has as one of its ideals the transformation of the hospital into the thank-you place.

One of the hospital's employee-related objectives is to avoid layoffs. The Williamsport Hospital & Medical Center is the only hospital in the region that has not laid off a single employee in the last 10 years and intends to make every effort to avoid layoffs in the future.

MAKING THE BUSINESS AND QUALITY SYNONYMOUS: Departmental Objectives Derived From Corporate Objectives

As we have already seen, the corporate staff envision the hospital's corporate business strategy and a commitment to continuous quality improvement to be one in the same thing. That is why the hospital's business objectives are quality objectives.

Our vice-president for business development, Jack Bustin, and our chief fiscal officer, Mike Scherneck, lend the influence of their perspectives and orientation to make this identification a pervasive mind set in how we plan and operationalize our business strategies.

Whenever I talk at other hospitals around the country, the question invariably comes up: "If you have so much training, don't you sometimes have to fill in for or pay overtime to employees in training? Doesn't that cost money?" Yes and yes. But Jack and Mike and Don Creamer and the rest of the corporate staff consider training to be an investment with a big payoff not an expenditure that just raises costs. So, the question I hear virtually everywhere never gets asked at home. That's something about which I am enormously grateful.

To make sure that this quality direction permeates the entire organization, every department must derive all of its objectives from the six corporate objectives of the hospital relating to:

- Customer service.
- Employee relations.
- Increased market share.
- Cost containment.
- Collaboration with physicians.
- A seamless delivery system for the era of managed care.

Here's how that works. One of the key items on which we are all evaluated are special projects. Special projects must all be related to our corporate objectives (see Resource 2-4). During my evaluation last year, *some* of the expectations Don Creamer and I agreed I'd work on in the fiscal year 1993–94 were:

- *Customer service*—Train all 1,500 employees in a program called "Quality C.A.R.E. in Trying Times—The Scoop."
- *Employee relations*—Work with the corporate staff and management staff to raise the hospital's employee climate assessment to above 90 percent.
- *Increased market share*—maintain the number of rehabilitation inpatients at 1992–93 levels (our Rehab. Center reports to me).
- *Cost containment*—Work with management team to eliminate 25 full-time positions without lay-offs.
- *Collaboration with physicians*—Deliver "the scoop" to the staff of our 80 employed physicians.
- *Seamless delivery system*—Provide occasional training to managers at hospitals likely to be part of our managed care network.

All of our corporate staff and department heads do the same sort of thing for their departments. During the annual evaluation interview, corporate staff members evaluate their department heads' success in achieving their previous year's corporate-derived departmental objectives and set new corporate-derived departmental objectives for the upcoming evaluation year. Department heads go through a similar process with their supervisors, and supervisors set out individual

---

Resource 2-4.   Examples of Achieved Corporate-Derived Departmental Goals

1. Customer service
    Emergency room: Reduce E.R. elopements from current rate of 70 a month (!) to no more and preferably less than 10 a month within 6 months.

2. Employee relations
    Demonstrate an increase in an Ancillary Department: Raise overall employee satisfaction ratings from 68 percent to at least 85 percent through a re-administration of our employee organizational climate assessment in nine months.

3. Increased market share
    Rehabilitation center: Increase admissions to the inpatient from the current rate of 28 a month to 40 a month in one year.

4. Cost containment
    Two nursing units: Eliminate $350,000 in labor costs without layoffs through the consolidation of two under-used medical/surgical nursing units.

5. Collaboration with physicians
    All departments: Earn a 95 percent satisfaction rating from our medical staff on our employees' collaboration with them in the care of their patients.

6. A seamless delivery system for managed care
    Hospital: Propose a business alliance with our principal competitor to provide more cost-efficient and high-quality care to our community.

---

employee expectations that are confined to the six areas of focus articulated in the hospital's overall objectives.

Through the annual performance evaluation process, the corporate staff ensures that all department activities and employee initiatives are consistent with true north—that is, the mission statement, the value statement, and the goals of the hospital. Employees and customers are all that matter—and no one should be involved in doing anything else but serving and exceeding their needs.

CARING FOR THE CAREGIVERS:
Regular Organizational Climate Assessments

In its relationship with hospital employees, the corporate staff has set standards for senior management performance, for departmental and supervisory performance, and for the maintenance of a work environment that is conducive to quality care (see Resource 2-5). These standards have been translated into a survey through which employees evaluate the hospital's managerial and organizational climate.

Items evaluating senior management include:

- The corporate staff runs this organization effectively.
- Overall hospital rules and policies make sense.
- The corporate staff is reasonably responsive to employee's needs and concerns.

Resource 2-5.   1991 Goals to Improve Organizational Climate

The Hospital has set the following five year hospitalwide goals:

1. Hospital wide overall target for positive ratings—90 percent.
2. All departments—a positive rating of 80% of more.
3. Up to 90 percent ASAP on the following items:
   - Recognition.
   - Value employees.
   - Input on decisions affecting employee work.
4. Blitz on:
   - Promotions.
   - Opportunities for growth and development.
   - Cooperation among departments.
5. Special department plans for improving employee relations
6. Human resources department/vice-president/department heads work on selected departments.

- Generally, The Williamsport Hospital & Medical Center is a safe place to work.
- The Williamsport Hospital responds positively and quickly to customer feedback.
- Employees here are expected to provide the very best in patient care.
- The Williamsport Hospital & Medical Center really values its employees.

Items evaluating department heads and supervisors include:

- Communication from our department head is frank and honest.
- The work rules and policies in my department make sense.
- The working conditions in our department are good.
- My supervisor recognizes me when I do a good job.
- Our supervisors are reasonably responsive to employee's needs and concerns.
- I feel free to discuss problems and concerns with my supervisor.
- The work rules and policies in my department are fairly administered.
- Employees here already have effective ways of bringing their suggestions and ideas to management's attention.

Items evaluating the overall climate include:

- Promotions here are based on merit and qualification.
- People in different departments cooperate well with each other.
- Overall, The Williamsport Hospital & Medical Center is a good place to work.
- My job is interesting and challenging.
- I receive the information I need to do my job properly.
- There are good opportunities to grow and advance here.
- Most people in our department get along well with each other.
- I feel pleased to work at The Williamsport Hospital & Medical Center.
- I have the tools and equipment to do my job properly.
- Employees in my department have adequate ways of expressing their views on decisions that affect them.

- I am proud to be an employee of The Williamsport Hospital & Medical Center.
- I would not have any reservations about having a member of my family cared for at The Williamsport Hospital & Medical Center.
- I would feel comfortable referring friends, neighbors, and community members to The Williamsport Hospital & Medical Center.
- The Williamsport Hospital & Medical Center is a better place to work than most other area organizations.
- The Williamsport Hospital is the best hospital in the region.

We have always thought that customer perception is the key criterion for measuring service quality. From the very beginning of our quality efforts we have also considered employee perceptions to be the principal criterion of the quality of the work environment at the Hospital. Consequently, we allow our regular organizational climate assessments to serve as employee report cards on the performance of our senior management and mid-level and supervisory managers and work to continuously improve the level of our performance in accordance with the feedback we receive from the employee group.

In chapter 8, we give a full description of how we conduct our organization climate assessments and implement recommendations based on the conclusions and analyses of these regularly administered questionnaires.

THE HOW-TO CQI KIT: The Williamsport Hospital & Medical Center's CQI Reference Manual

Over the past decade, several organizations have formed to have English declared the one and only official language in the United States. Among other things, they would like to see English as the only language used in the public schools. These organizations reflect the view that a common required language unifies people and creates solidarity and community among people of diverse backgrounds. There's also another side to this debate. Opponents of this view do not deny the unifying potency of a common language, but they do contend that this route to unity smothers and sacrifices the kind of enriching diversity characteristic of vibrant societies.

Gratefully, the call for a common CQI vocabulary does not provoke this kind of controversy. At The Williamsport Hospital & Medical Center, we have staff on both sides of the societal debate who concur that a singularly defined vocabulary facilitates understanding and cooperation. Therefore, at The Williamsport Hospital & Medical Center we have felt a similar need to draw our many different employees together in a united pursuit of service excellence.

The hospital's CQI manual is the definitive resource that describes in detail, the what, the why, and the how of continuous quality improvement at The Williamsport Hospital & Medical Center.

The CQI resource manual was put together so that everyone working on improvement projects had a common and consistent guide to The Williamsport Hospital & Medical Center's preferred method for planning, conducting, integrating, and implementing continuous quality improvement. The manual enables newly formed teams to speak the same quality language, begin from the same quality assumptions, use the same quality process, and bring completed projects from the study phase to the implementation and evaluation phase.

The CQI manual is divided into the following chapters:

- *Section 1.* Corporate Goals
- *Section 2.* CQI—The Big Picture
- *Section 3.* QA vs. QI
- *Section 4.* General CQI Overview
- *Section 5.* The "How To" for CQI
- *Section 6.* CQI Tools
- *Section 7.* Teamwork
- *Section 8.* Resources
- *Section 9.* Statistics
- *Section 10.* Existing Teams
- *Section 11.* Glossary

(See Resource 2-C in the Appendix for a complete outline.)

HOW TO MANAGE KEY MOMENTS OF TRUTH:
The Quality Service Plan

Six years ago, the hospital conducted a course called "Nuts and Bolts of Service Management I" based on *Service America* (Dow-Jones Irwin, 1985), by Ron Zemke and Karl Albrecht. During the six, two-hour sessions all of the management staff learned how to develop departmental and interdepartmental quality service plans describing:

- All their customers.
- Each customer's expectation for each moment of truth in the service cycle.
- Each department's plan for developing a distinctive service strategy and a system responsive to the service quality expectations of all its customers. Each department completes a refined version of the plan every year. Over 200 of our 1,500 employees participate in this formal ongoing improvement, and many others contribute ideas for the annual updates.

The quality service plan contains literally hundreds of moments of truth we strive to transform into magic moments. See Resource 2-6 for a sample departmental service plan in our recovery room and Resource 2-D in the Appendix for a sample departmental service plan for anesthesiology.

"Nuts and Bolts of Service Management I" is offered every year and the hospital's more than 300-page plan for service excellence is updated annually by each department within the hospital.

KEEPING IT ALL TOGETHER: The MEDIMPROVE Committee

A favorite tool of CQI practitioners is statistical process control (SPC). It is ironic that in our enthusiasm to make sure that processes throughout our organizations are in control, we are oblivious to the fact that the CQI process itself is often the process most out of control. CQI teams may be working on customer encounters, service systems or processes, or healthcare pathways that do not correspond to high-priority

Resource 2-6. Quality Service Plan			
Customer	**Moment of Truth**	**Customer Expectation/Needs**	**Service Plan (Who, What, When, Where, How)**
Physician	(M1) Greeting in recovery room	(1) Courteous greeting, acknowledgement ofhis or her presence. Information about patient's location.	*Who:* R.N. and Unit Clerk *What:* Provide attention and direction to the physician. *When:* As soon as M.D. enters the recovery room. *Where:* Recovery Room. *How:* Greet M.D. in friendly way with his last name. Direct him to patient's bedside. Unit Clerk will act as liaison to direct M.D.
	(M2) Personal contact	(2) Location of information regarding patient's condition.	*Who:* R.N. *What:* Provide information to M.D. *When:* As soon as M.D. comes into recovery room proper. *Where:* recovery room. *How:* Greet in friendly manner.
	(M3) Telephone call	(3) Prompt and friendly greeting. Pertinent information available.	Organize information and questions. Communicate information to another R.N. if assigned R.N. away from recovery room.

customer needs. Teams may be floundering because they have no trained facilitator. Teams may be misusing or inappropriately use CQI tools. CQI studies may not get implemented and evaluated. CQI teams may proliferate, procrastinate, obfuscate, and intimidate—everything but ameliorate. No one is in control.

Our MEDIMPROVE committee principal function is to make sure all of our CQI efforts are focused on the right things, done in the right way, and phased over time to allow our quality improvement projects to be models of quality themselves. Positions represented on the MED-IMPROVE committee are:

- Chairmen: Steve Johnson, Executive Vice-President/Chief Operating Officer, and Joseph English, M.D., Vice-President/Medical Director
- Marcie Finn, M.D., Chairperson, Patient Care Committee
- Gregory Frailey, D.O., Medical Director, Ambulatory Care Services
- Dan Glunk, M.D., Employed Physician
- William McClain, Vice-President/Marketing
- Jack Bustin, Vice-President/Planning and Business Development
- Jeannie Hill, Vice-President/Clinical Services
- Tim Mannello, Vice-President/Human Resources
- Candy Dewar, Assistant Vice-President/Nursing
- Linda Boose, Director of Physician Office Practices
- Bob Ireland, Director of Management Engineering/Facilitator Training
- Robert Wallace, Director of Risk Management/MEDIMPROVE Project Coordinator
- Barbara Proffitt, Quality Assessment Supervisor
- Rosanne Mattiace, Patient Care Manager, ICU
- Jeffrey Wetstone, M.D., Program Director, Family Practice Residency Program

Each year, the MEDIMPROVE committee processes about 15 to 20 cycle of service projects, about 50 departmental CQI submissions to the Chairman's Quality Award Program and 10 to 20 clinical pathway projects. Resource 2-7 contains examples of past and current projects that will give a flavor of the kind of CQI projects the committee typically monitors.

Resource 2-7. Sample Projects Completed in 1993-94

C.A.R.E. Dimension
Chaplaincy

Project Title	Work Areas Involved	Desired Outcomes
Chaplaincy Care Competencies	Clinical Pastoral Education students, Chaplain volunteer visitors; Chaplain on-call volunteer	High level of respect expressed for patient and family beliefs; timeliness of chaplain visits

Ambulatory Care Services

Project Title	Work Areas Involved	Desired Outcomes
Healthy Beginnings Plus Program Improvements	Family planning; Birthplace; Life center; Ambulatory care clinic; Family practice; Community relations; Social services	Increased volumes; greater patient satisfaction; increased awareness of services; improved infant care; improved patient environment

TQM
4 East, 3 East, 4 West, ICU, Emergency Services

Project Title	Work Areas Involved	Desired Outcomes
Patient Admission from ER to Units	ER, 4 East, 3 East, ICU, 4 West	Patient transfer to room in acceptable time; appropriate report from ER to unit; preparation on unit; increased trust

Resource 2-7.   Sample Projects Completed in 1993-94 *(continued)*

Surgical Services

Project Title	Work Areas Involved	Desired Outcomes
OR Turn-Around time	OR staff; Anesthesia staff; Environmental services	Higher compared to national averages; specific time based on specialty; improved booking

MEDIMPROVE
Pharmacy

Project Title	Work Areas Involved	Desired Outcomes
The Expedient Conversion of Intravenous Medications to the Least Invasive Therapy	Pharmacy, Nursing, Gastroenterology; Infectious disease	Eliminate delays in conversion; develop protocols for pharmacist and nurses; decreased cost

Anesthesia

Project Title	Work Areas Involved	Desired Outcomes
Anesthesia Preop Process, Revisited	Medical departments of surgery and anesthesia, hospital departments of anesthesia and surgical services; Pre-admission testing	Improve process and content of anesthesia workup; reduce lab work pre-op; cost controls

Here are some sample current projects:

- Standard format for patient management guidelines—undergoing a 6-month in-house test.
- Benchmark studies on congestive heart failure with six other hospitals in the Voluntary Hospitals of America network.
- Patient satisfaction survey for the hospital's Rehabilitation Center.
- Transient Ischemic Attack Practice Management Guidelines.
- Annual Update of Service Quality Plan.
- MEDIMPROVE Plan for 1993-94.

People make quality happen. Structures and institutionally integrated practices make quality last. At The Williamsport Hospital & Medical Center, those supporting institutional practices include a repetitive, unchanging and challenging quality message, a board whose principal responsibility is to ensure quality to the community, a corporate staff that leads the operational aspects of CQI, a management team accountable for implementing quality initiatives, a market research capacity that keeps our understanding of customer needs current and accurate, a universally understood, three-dimensional customer-focused definition of quality and quality criteria, a value inspiring C.A.R.E. for employees and customers to see our business as quality, an evaluative role and mechanism for our employees, a Quality How-To Kit, a Quality Game Plan, and a group of involved people to pull and keep it all together.

The MEDIMPROVE Committee coordinates many CQI initiatives during the year. To ensure adequate attention to all of the improvement projects conducted throughout the Hospital, the MEDIMPROVE Committee establishes reporting schedules for the year and revises the schedules as unplanned but necessary projects are planned and implemented. For example, the MEDIMPROVE Committee's Reporting Schedule for 1993 is given in Table 2.1.

TABLE 2.1 CQI REPORTING SCHEDULE TO THE MEDIMPROVE COMMITTEE: 1993

	Jan	Feb	Mar	Apr	May	June	July	Aug	Sept	Oct	Nov	Dec
CARE	X	X	X	X	X	X	X	X	X	X	X	X
MEDIMPROVE (3 reports on required format*)												
(examples—CHF, CVA, Rehab, Knees/Hips/Chemo)												
CHAIRMAN'S Quality Award Summary Report					X							
Cycle of Service Teams (Annually)												
—Outpatient Diagnostic and Therapy Patients												
—Cancer Care Patients												
—Same Day Surgery Patients												
—Inpatient Elective Admissions												
—Cardiac Surgery Quality Task Force												
—Emergency Room Quality Management Team "A"												
—Emergency Room Quality Management Team "B"												
HOSPITAL DATA BASE REVIEW (Semi-Annually)												
—MedisGroups/Atlas			X						X			
—FIMS (Functional Impact Measurement Studies)				X						X		
—Tumor Registry					X						X	
—ORSOS						X						X
SATISFACTION SURVEYS (Patient/Physician)	X		X		X		X		X		X	
SENTINEL EVENTS (Monitoring and Evaluation) (Semi-Annually)												
—JCAHO Recommended Indicators												

TABLE 2.1   CQI REPORTING SCHEDULE TO THE MEDIMPROVE COMMITTEE: 1993 (*continued*)

	Jan	Feb	Mar	Apr	May	June	July	Aug	Sept	Oct	Nov	Dec
OB/PEDS				X						X		
ANESTHESIA	X						X					
—Medical Staff Departments (attached)					X						X	
—Medical Staff Committees (attached)						X						X
—Clinical Departments (1st split)— including Quality Control (attached)		X						X				
—Clinical Departments (2nd split)— including Quality Control (attached)			X						X			

*Format
1—Situation Analysis
2—Goals/Recommendations
3—Results

Medical Staff Departments (May, November)
  —Anesthesia
  —Ambulatory Care
  —Family Practice
  —Medicine
  —OB/GYN
  —Pathology
  —Pediatrics
  —Physical Medicine & Rehabilitation
  —Psychiatry
  —Radiology
  —Surgery

Medical Staff Committees (June, December)
  —Tissue and Transfusion
  —ICU
  —CCU
  —Medical Records

TABLE 2.1   CQI REPORTING SCHEDULE TO THE MEDIMPROVE COMMITTEE: 1993 (*continued*)

—P&T—DUE
—Infection Control
—Cancer

Clinical Departments—1st split (February, August)
—Nursing
—Surgical Services
—Laboratory
—Social Services
—Dietary
—Pharmacy

Clinical Departments—2nd split (March, September)
—Ambulatory Care (including Ambulatory Care Clinic, Family Practice and Paramedics)
—Radiology
—Sports Medicine
—PM&R
—H&L Center
—Nuclear Medicine
—Psychology

3

Setting and Communicating Quality Standards

"There are two kinds of people in the world: People who get things done and people who take credit for it. Strive to be a member of the first group: there's less competition."

—Indira Ghandi

It was no way to start the afternoon of my first day at work at The Williamsport Hospital & Medical Center. Three very upset nurses came to my office alleging they had witnessed a transport orderly "roughly plop" a very sick elderly gentleman on a litter. My boss, Don Creamer, came to my office just after I had completed a separate interview with each of the nurses, received their written statements of complaint, met with the employee in question, and talked to our labor relations attorney. I told Don what had happened and that I was convinced that what the nurses charged was absolutely true. He asked me what I intended to do. I said that we intended to terminate the young man effective the next day. "No," Don responded, "Have him clear his locker right now, tell him that he is not welcome on this campus and that he should only return when he has business and with permission from Charlie Wolverton, in safety and security." The Williamsport Hospital & Medical Center's official customer quality standard had been established before a written or verbal standard was ever promulgated.

If standards are to carry any weight, they are not merely set down and communicated in writing. They are lived out in daily practice.

Violations of quality standards are not tolerated, and performance that exceeds standards is fostered and rewarded. For example, as we shall see later, every department in the hospital must develop and implement a CQI project that corresponds to a high-quality need in one of the dimensions of quality. For the fifth year in a row, we have visibly rewarded departments whose submissions were deemed best against specific criteria. This year, our MEDIMPROVE committee required four departments to do their submissions over because they did not meet minimum requirements. Our training standards require participants to master and apply defined managerial skills. At the end of our training programs, managers must take a combination written and oral exam. Some fail.

The imperative to treat our customers like gold is effectively conveyed when we, for example, honor and reward our C.A.R.E. stars and swiftly and strenuously deal with employees whose behavior toward our patients or employees is personally or professionally unacceptable or offensive. So, over the last nine years we have honored more than 200 C.A.R.E. employees of the month, 18 C.A.R.E. employees of the year, 50 physicians of the month, 6 physicians of the year, and more than 10,000 magic moment makers who have transformed moments of truth into go-beyond customer service encounters.

We have also terminated more than 200 employees, including seven for sexual harassment and four for verbally abusing a patient. Six years ago, we lost close to 300 admissions a year when we confronted a physician about harassing one of our employees (good riddance as far as we were concerned). We do not actively recruit physicians to become our employees. Yet since this event, the size of our employed physician group has doubled to about 100 physicians. This increase has more than compensated for the lost admissions. We can't measure the positive effect of the action on our employees' motivation and morale. Suffice it to say that the episode demonstrated more convincingly that we really care for our employees than does our frequent communication of the fact.

The tools for setting and communicating standards of quality described in the rest of this chapter are just that—tools. If they are consistently supported and implemented with the managerial resolve that translates them into standard operating procedure, places that are really serious about their standards end up having more people who get the work done than who are merely looking to get credit for it.

QUALITY EXPECTATIONS DEFINE QUALITY RESULTS:
Measurable Performance Evaluations

People give you what you expect—at least more often than not. Studies in occupational and educational settings have repeatedly shown that
individuals of roughly equal competence produce far superior results in
similarly controlled circumstances when they are challenged by goals
that exceed their reach. That's why in getting people started toward the
achievement of our customer- and employee-related standards, we
work with every employee to set realistic but challenging work expectations or goals. In the framework of Ken Blanchard's ABCs of management, the *A* stands for activation through goal setting. Together with
our employees we set out job expectations for an evaluation in three
aspects of their work.

Job responsibilities as contained
in an updated job description

Here our supervisors and employees jointly define specific expectations for their technical and professional performance. For example,
my own job description includes the following item: "Assist management in creating and maintaining an organizational climate that
enhances the effective delivery of quality services." Consequently, my
annual performance review focuses on the year's hospitalwide and
departmental organizational climate assessments. In the case of our
caregivers, these expectations relate directly to their responsibility for
delivering favorable healthcare outcomes—what we refer to as MED-
IMPROVE—the clinical and medical dimension of quality.

Special quality-related projects
for the evaluation period

Each employee has the responsibility of making our services better in
the year ahead than they were in the past evaluation year. Here we
jointly define personal areas for quality improvement in one or more of
the three dimensions of quality for the following year. Special projects
must derive from, complement, and support one or more of our six

corporate objectives. Last year for example, because quality employees are a prerequisite to quality services, one of my 10 assigned special projects was to train and monitor human resources staff as they applied screening techniques on customer relations skills with presenting employment candidates.

Interpersonal and managerial performance

The dimension of quality that individual employees can most directly affect is their interpersonal relationships with our patients and other customers and with their fellow employees, and in the case of our managers, our supervisory relationships with our colleagues and associates. Here we define the detailed C.A.R.E. behaviors that employees are expected to practice in their relationships with patients and guests; others in their department, including their supervisors; employees in other departments; and physicians. For example, our medical director, Joe English, M.D., like all of our managers, deals directly with any member of the medical staff whose behavior is incompatible with our patient care and employee relations culture. A year or so ago, Joe worked through a remarkable transformation with a physician notorious for unprofessional outbursts of temper.

In our mandatory basic leadership course for supervisors, managers learn that regular verbal feedback on the results of one's work in each of the three dimensions of quality is the most important part of a manager's evaluative responsibilities. They learn to intervene with positive feedback when possible and with constructive corrective feedback when necessary. In a separate session of that course, managers are taught the purpose, characteristics, and methods for conducting what we like to call our annual appreciation review, the measurable performance evaluation. (Resource 3-A in the Appendix shows our general directions for conducting such a review.)

THE PROFESSIONAL STANDARD OF CONDUCT:
25 C.A.R.E. Behaviors

Some of the most eternally grateful, satisfied customers our hospital has are family members of patients who have died. Although a reliable favorable medical outcome is still *the* most important dimension of hospital quality, in the real world, patients and their family members and visitors largely evaluate the quality of an institution like a hospital by the way they were treated. And the small, thoughtful, personal, and special things done for them by people throughout a hospital are largely what people talk about after an admission. For most patients, the quality of the interpersonal interactions with employees is an important cue of quality. Personal treatment is about the only dimension of quality care that every patient can accurately evaluate. The next time someone describes a hospital experience they've had, notice the words they use. When things go right, they usually say things like: "The nurses were great." "The employees were friendly." "Everybody really cared." When a patient is displeased, we hear these kinds of refrains: "The brown haired lab tech on at night was rude." "It took forever to get my bell answered." "No one ever took enough time to explain things to me."

What do employees have to do, you ask, to earn the respect of patients and other customers as service providers who: do their utmost to get the job done right the first time (reliability), give the appearance of professionals (tangibles), instill confidence in patients (reassurance), get on things quickly and see them through (responsiveness), and do things as if there were no one more special than the customer at hand (empathy)? In answering that question, we did not start from scratch. Instead, we adopted and adapted the C.A.R.E. behaviors in what we consider to be a well-defined customer relations package, the C.A.R.E. Program developed a decade ago in the Midwest by Personal and Professional Development, Inc. (In this instance, C.A.R.E. stands for courtesy, attitude, respect, and empathy.)

Starting with our original kickoff quality training and running throughout our training ever since, the 25 C.A.R.E. behaviors (see Resource 3-1) have been an important element of the behavioral expectations we have attempted to inculcate in our employees. From the very beginning, these C.A.R.E. behaviors have been a formal part of our ongoing regular feedback and an explicit element in our annual appreciation reviews. We select our C.A.R.E. employees of the month and our C.A.R.E. employees and physician of the year on the basis of the 25 C.A.R.E. behaviors. In our minds, these 25 C.A.R.E. behaviors constitute the behavioral expression of the C.A.R.E. ideal. You can tell

---

Resource 3-1.   C.A.R.E. Behaviors

1) Acknowledges and greets visitors, patients, and co-workers whenever he/she meets them.

2) Responds to patients, visitors, and fellow workers in a pleasant, respectful, and professional way.

3) Anticipates the needs of visitors, patients, and peers and helps them out whenever possible.

4) Introduces self, mentions his/her department or position, explains functions he/she is there to perform.

5) Answers the inquiries of patients, guests, and co-workers *(especially new employees)* in a patient, helpful, and positive way.

6) Obtains information or refers guests to proper source when unable to provide an answer.

7) Opens doors, holds open elevator doors for people wheeling carts or carrying things.

8) Practices listening and identifying skills when guests *(whether patient or visitor)* get upset.

9) Makes a special effort to practice C.A.R.E. surface skills the first time he/she meets a patient, guest, or co-worker.

10) Maintains a neat, well-groomed, and professional appearance that creates a positive image for The Williamsport Hospital & Medical Center.

11) Does his/her part in keeping the hospital clean *(not leaving mess; picks up after self; picks up debris).*

12) Demonstrates concern for the rights, privacy, and feelings of patients, guests, and co-workers.

13) Interacts with others in a businesslike, professional manner; avoids idle conversation that excludes guests.

14) When time allows, answers phone this way:

—*(Greeting)* Hello

—*(Department)* Maintenance

—*(Name optional)* John Moore *(speaking)*

—*(Climate Setter)* May I help you?

15) Demonstrates concern for confidentiality of patient information when talking with the patient or when in public areas.

16) Treats hospital patients and visitors as guests to our "home."

Resource 3-1.   C.A.R.E. Behaviors *(continued)*

---

17) Explains reasons for our rules, regulations, and policies when asked to do so by patients and visitors.

18) Keeps his/her work environment neat and professional looking at all times.

19) Shows pride, interest, and enthusiasm in his/her work.

20) Goes out of his/her way to recognize everyone he/she meets as an individual person.

21) Tries to be the kind of person others would like to work with.

22) Interacts with co-workers to help promote good working relationships.

23) Treats all employees regardless of department or position with dignity and respect.

24) Is in the habit of "helping out" fellow-workers whenever he/she can.

25) Shows pride in The Williamsport Hospital & Medical Center *(together we are The Williamsport Hospital & Medical Center)*.

---

who genuinely embodies a C.A.R.E.ing attitude by these clearly defined and readily observable external behavioral manifestations.

THE MANAGER'S CODE OF CONDUCT:
Leadership C.A.R.E. Pledge

Do unto your employees as you would have them do unto your customers. That sentiment goes back at least as far as the hey-day of the young Bill Marriott, founder of the Marriott Hotel chain. If the 25 C.A.R.E. behaviors are a sure-fire way to make your patients and other customers feel they've been on the receiving end of go-beyond quality, we think that the 10 behaviors contained in our adaptation of the Marriott Leadership Pledge (see Resource 3-2) provide a fail-safe blueprint for motivating and empowering employees to provide it.

Funny how seminars on quality always emphasize what employees need to do for customers and seldom dwell at length on what managers

---

Resource 3-2.   The Leadership C.A.R.E. Pledge

I PROMISE THE MEMBERS OF MY TEAM, THAT AS I FULFILL MY RESPONSIBILITY TO ENSURE THE DELIVERY OF GO-BEYOND QUALITY TO ALL OUR CUSTOMERS I WILL STRIVE TO:

1. *SET AN EXAMPLE OF COURTESY, ATTENTIVENESS, RESPONSIVENESS, EMPATHY (C.A.R.E.) FOR THEM BY MY OWN ACTIONS IN ALL THINGS.*
2. *MAINTAIN AN APPROACHABLE AND OPEN ATTITUDE TO ENCOURAGE GOOD COMMUNICATIONS AND TO FOSTER A SUPPORTIVE WORK ENVIRONMENT.*
3. *ACT FAIRLY IMPARTIALLY, AND CONSISTENTLY IN MATTERS RELATING TO WORK RULES, DISCIPLINE, AND REWARDS.*
4. *SHOW A SINCERE, PERSONAL INTEREST IN THEM AS INDIVIDUALS WITHOUT BECOMING OVERLY FAMILIAR.*
5. *SEEK THEIR COUNSEL ON MATTERS THAT AFFECT THEIR JOBS AND BE GUIDED AS MUCH AS POSSIBLE BY THEIR JUDGMENT.*
6. *ALLOW THEM AS MUCH INDIVIDUALITY AS POSSIBLE IN THE WAY THEIR JOBS ARE PERFORMED, AS LONG AS THE QUALITY OF THE RESULT AND THE QUALITY OF THEIR RELATIONSHIPS WITH ALL ARE NOT COMPROMISED.*
7. *MAKE SURE THEY ALWAYS KNOW IN ADVANCE WHAT I EXPECT FROM THEM WITH REGARD TO THEIR CONDUCT AND PERFORMANCE ON THE JOB.*
8. *DEMONSTRATE REGULARLY MY APPRECIATION OF THEIR EFFORTS AND EXPRESS PRAISE TO THEM FOR THEIR ACCOMPLISHMENTS.*
9. *USE EVERY OPPORTUNITY TO TEACH THEM HOW TO DO THEIR JOBS BETTER AND HOW TO HELP THEMSELVES ADVANCE IN SKILL LEVEL AND RESPONSIBILITY.*
10. *SHOW THEM THAT I CAN "DO" AS WELL AS "MANAGE" BY PITCHING IN TO WORK BESIDE THEM WHEN MY HELP IS NEEDED.*

SIGNED _____

WITNESS _____

need to do for employees to lead employees to want to deliver quality. The impression is that the only relationship that needs to be managed in total quality management is the relationship between the service provider and the external customer. But that's not so. As it is often taught, total quality management isn't total at all. Too often, too many have too little to say about the second relationship that needs to be managed when TQM is totally implemented: the relationship between service managers and service providers. Managers or leaders in business settings are responsible for results—results that are largely achieved through the efforts of others. Getting people to want to and to be able to deliver services that surpass customer expectations is the bottomline result for which managers ought be held accountable above all else in a TQM setting.

At The Williamsport Hospital & Medical Center, each year we ask every corporate staff member, every department head, and every supervisor to sign the hospital's leadership C.A.R.E. pledge and to have the pledge witnessed by his or her supervisor. We have printed the pledge on embossed paper and have had it framed so that our supervisors can keep the pledge in their offices as a reminder of their responsibilities and obligations to our employees in their effort to achieve go-beyond quality. Supervisors see the leadership C.A.R.E. pledge as a public manifestation of expectations that have been in place and monitored for years; employees, as a sign that the hospital promises to care for them regardless of who is a member of the management team in the future. Our corporate staff thinks of the pledge as one more tangible sign that those who come on in a leadership capacity at our hospital must conform to our C.A.R.E. culture and not try to change that culture to be compatible with any of their own contrary predilections.

We have also enlarged this leadership C.A.R.E. pledge into a 36-inch-by-18-inch velox and then each year, we have every member of the management staff from the corporate level to the supervisory level sign this enlarged version of the pledge. We then frame it and hang it in the cafeteria to remind our employees of our continuing commitment to support their efforts to provide quality C.A.R.E. to our patients and other customers. Visitors are astonished and impressed by the display. Supervisors and employees think of the display as just a reminder of expectations long in place. Most important, no one sees the display as a gimmick because it is a *public* expression of an existing reality and not a hollow promise contradicted by daily practice.

ON NOT HIDING ONE'S LIGHT UNDER A BUSHEL:
10 Commandments of Service

The real is not always clearly visible. In the physical realm, you can't always see threats to your well-being at work in the dark. Remember the terrifying cellar scene in the film *Silence of the Lambs* when the heroine was literally completely in the dark but her demented stalker saw her every move through infrared glasses. Remember similar images of American troops in Desert Storm peering out into the vast dark desert waste-lands from their tanks, their enemy illuminated as if it were daylight through the use of the same kind of equipment.

Years ago, I went to a large city hospital to receive treatment for a corneal ulcer. When I got to the ophthalmology reception desk, the receptionist continued her paperwork for five minutes before she looked up and said "Yes?" verbally and "What do *you* want?" nonverbally. Not only did she seem displeased that *I* was there, but she seemed none-too-thrilled to be there herself. A physician assistant hardly said a word as he did a perfunctory exam of my eye and vision. The surgeon could have been a before ad for a Dale Carnegie Course. My final impression: the irritated look on the face of the clerk when I said *her* choice of the date for *my* appointment was not convenient. My personal physician had told me that this was *the* place to go for my eye. If seeing is believing, I thought at the time, I would have to take my physician's recommendation on faith.

Quality, real quality, is sometimes like that—unobservable and unperceived because of the way our customers customarily look at things. In his popular work on paradigms, Joel Barker points out that we sometimes misinterpret reality because we impose our mind set and preconceptions on it. In a short interesting study in Karl Albrecht's book, *The Code of Quality Service,* he explains that Americans have a very set and restricted mind set about the external manifestations of any quality service. We often fail to appreciate the value of a job well done if the person doing the job fails to do certain definable things beyond doing the job right the first time. Just as infrared glasses enable us to see objects in the dark, so too the behaviors contained in the 10 commandments of quality service enable customers to see the reality of quality to which they would otherwise be blinded.

At the hospital where I worked 10 years ago, there were two surgeons whom the staff in the operating room considered were both among the very best—indistinguishably competent in their specialty. The one surgeon was always booked for months in advance; the other mostly picked up the emergency overflow. The difference: without knowing it, the first surgeon was a natural practitioner of the 10 commandments of quality service outlined below. The second—the very antithesis.

When properly and consistently executed, the 25 C.A.R.E. behaviors, the Leadership C.A.R.E. Pledge, our CQI system improvements, our MEDIMPROVE clinical pathways, and our service quality plan constitute the reality of quality which we provide daily. Dr. Albrecht argues that many of our customers will be oblivious to these accomplishments if they are not illuminated by the universal and consistent demonstration of these simple but telling behaviors:

- Rule 1: Greet guests immediately.
- Rule 2: Give guests your undivided attention.
- Rule 3: Make the first 30 seconds count.
- Rule 4: Be natural, not phony or mechanical.
- Rule 5: Be enthusiastic and cordial.
- Rule 6: Be the guest's problem-solver.
- Rule 7: Think. Use your common sense when ordinary procedures aren't enough.
- Rule 8: Within reason, bend the rules when necessary.
- Rule 9: Make the last 30 seconds count.
- Rule 10: Be up. Stay up. Take good care of yourself.

The 25 C.A.R.E. behaviors are the behaviors that constitute the meat, the substance, the reality of the first dimension of quality just-as-you-like-it personal service. They are the what of dimension 1 of quality. The ten commandments of quality service are the infrared glasses that enable customers to perceive the what of quality in all three dimensions of quality: the personal service dimension, the systems dimension, and the healthcare dimension.

As we have seen, total quality management involves the management of two relationships: the relationship between our employees and customers and the relationship between our managers and our employees. By the same token, total quality management involves the management of the reality of quality—that is, the quality of personal interactions, service systems, and the medical outcomes and procedures of our care. Total quality management also involves the management or the illumination of the customer's perception of quality to ensure that the quality service objectively rendered and received is subjectively perceived and appreciated. We constantly strive to illuminate the perception of our customers to the quality we offer as a matter of practice by promoting the constant practice of the 10 commandments by all of our employees. We educate our customers to expect treatment in accordance with these 10 commandments through plaques summarizing them called Our Quality Promise To You (see Resource 3-3). The plaques are highly visible in locations throughout the institution.

SATURATING THE AIRWAYS:
Go-Beyond Quality Is All That Matters

There's an old Latin saying: *"Repetitio mater studiorum."* Literally, the saying means repetition is the mother of studies or more freely, repetition is the mother of learning. Repetition, we've come to see, is also the mother of all effective organizational communication. We try to repeat what it is we stand for every chance we get: at our recognition dinners, at our C.A.R.E. employee of the month lunches and C.A.R.E. employees of the year banquet, at our president's four open forums every year, in all of our orientation and training programs, at our weekly department head meetings, at our management meetings, during our management development courses, in our policy manual, in our employee manual, in our weekly newsletter, in everything we communicate by word or action to our employees.

The task of an effective leader is not simply to communicate an institution's values and goals but to ensure that they are assimilated and executed. At home, at work, everywhere, employees are constantly bombarded with the message: the only thing that is constant is change. But with quality, there are some rock-bottom beliefs that will last, some principles that never change:

- Quality is the competitive edge.
- Quality is our business strategy.

Resource 3-3. Commandments Summary Plaque

❖

QUALITY SERVICE:
OUR PROMISE TO YOU

Our highest priority is to provide you with quality service.
As patients and guests of The Williamsport Hospital & Medical Center,
you have every right to expect:

❖ A courteous greeting and a smile.
❖ The complete attention of the employees serving you.
❖ Careful consideration of your special needs.
❖ People who can identify with your situation.
❖ An empathetic and responsive attitude.
❖ Respect and dignity while you are here.

Courtesy • Attentiveness • Responsiveness • Empathy

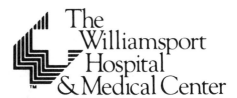

The Williamsport Hospital & Medical Center

© 1988 by The Williamsport Hospital & Medical Center

- The customer is the final arbiter of what quality is.
- Successful quality efforts never lose their customer focus.
- Winners in the quality sweepstakes focus limited resources on only the very, very most important and urgent customer priorities.
- The only correct response to the most extremely important high-priority customer needs is go-beyond quality.
- The link between customers' expectations and go-beyond quality is a workforce united in the pursuit of service excellence.
- Customers evaluate us on three dimensions of quality: personal service, user-friendly systems, and healthcare outcomes and procedures.
- Successful businesses institutionally integrate practices and policies that ensure the support of quality efforts in each of the three dimensions of quality.
- There should be continuity and openness to integrating new perspectives and tools in any conceptualization of CQI.

These truths, we believe, never change and need to be repeated, and repeated, and repeated.

As Viktor E. Frankl has said, "Man is an animal in search of meaning." All the victims of the horrors of the holocaust had, he said, one thing in common. They continued to hold on to the belief that there is some kind of meaning or purpose in life. You've got to believe in something that lasts if you are to remain motivated in persisting in the face of the most daunting experience like imprisonment in a death camp or in our less horrifying world, to contribute your best effort over the long term to a hospital's customer-focused value. People do not commit themselves to free-floating change, only to change they perceive to be a genuine improvement. Changes that improve things are marked by some unalterable characteristics and values. If quality is to take hold in an organization, these values must be constantly repeated.

ALIGNING PERSONAL AND PROFESSIONAL ASPIRATIONS WITH ORGANIZATIONAL QUALITY IDEALS:
What's In It for Me?

Motivation is an internal drive to achieve a goal in order to satisfy a need. We agree to doing the family's grocery shopping because we love to eat, forego spending money on frivolous items to buy our families the necessities of life, and join social groups because they make us feel that we belong. We work hard to do a job right because we need to know that what we do really counts.

The same line of reasoning applies in motivating employees toward quality goals. Quality efforts endure only as long as the achievement of quality goals promotes the achievement of personal and professional needs and aspirations. Challenging the employees in an institution to become a world-class act is no trivial thing. It is a call to exceed the merely passable and to consistently put forth a discretionary effort that differentiates outstanding services from those that are merely run of the mill. But why should an employee voluntarily try as hard as he or she can when in most places far less will do? And how can managers encourage their employees without manipulating them or bribing them through monetary incentives that soon lose their motivating force, cost the institution more than it can afford, and immediately get entrenched as an entitlement? How do we get employees to engage themselves as enthusiastically and intently in providing other people with service as they do in coaching soccer teams, leading girl and boy scout troops, and working for all kinds of other charitable organizations?

The call to quality is a challenge to change an employee's life in a place where he or she spends half of his or her waking hours. We at The Williamsport Hospital & Medical Center think motives that drive employees to go the extra mile outside work have application in the work setting as well. To help people in Abraham Lincoln's phrase, "Be touched by the better angels of their nature" when they are at work, we have employed two basic strategies:

- We appeal to the basic human needs that impel people to such generous involvement outside of work.
- We have made practical applications of what motivational theorists have had to say about workers as people.

First, emphasize three personal motivators as quality motivators. In all of our training, in fresh new ways, we frequently unveil this hidden but genuine alignment between our institution's quality goals and our employees' personal and professional aspirations through these three appeals:

- The only perspective from which we can accurately gauge the relative importance of the things that go on daily in our lives is the imagined perspective of the moment of our own death: The insight of hindsight. At that moment, what will be most significant is not the price of the house that we live in, the kind of car we drive, or all of the material possessions we've worked so hard to acquire. What will be important at that moment will be how we treated people: our spouse, our children, our parents, our family, our friends, those we meet every day, and the patients whose privilege it is for us to serve. That's what will be important. Unlike many others, people who work in hospitals have the opportunity to live out the innermost meaning of their human existence every day when they come to work.
- Everyone we meet in our call to serve is unique, special, unduplicatable, and unclonable in our never-to-be repeated existence, and each deserves our very best. Each is as distinctly different as the architectural design of every snowflake in a winter's blizzard, as unique as a fingerprint, a person's voice modulation, and as we've discovered through recent improvements in lab technology, as unique as every single person's blood. Each of our patients is as important and as special as we are and therefore merits the best that is in us to give.
- To a large extent, we *are* what we make and what we do. The products and services of our hands are a strong reflection of our inner worth. We are all part of a national movement to restore ourselves to the pride of our heritage: a pride in the words "Made by Me" and in the label "Made in the USA." As all sectors of our economy strive to reinvigorate our competitiveness in international markets, we are a small but significant part of that national effort. Especially within the broader context of our nation's struggle to restore our heritage, legacy, tradition, and challenge to quality, we frequently repeat the adage: "Don't leave the most important part out of q-ality."

The second basic strategy we at The Williamsport Hospital & Medical Center employ to sustain our employees' pursuits of the quality ideal is the application of the basic insights of motivational theory (Resource 3-B in the Appendix summarizes the principles of motivational theory):

- The platinum rule. Do unto others as they would have you do unto them—*not* do unto others as you would have them do unto you. At any particular time, different people are often motivated by different things. At different times, the same people are often motivated by different things. Many times, most people are motivated by the same things. Motivational strategies, therefore, must be targeted at individuals as well as at groups.
- Motivate people by appealing to their unmet needs (Abraham Maslow.) Don't appeal to already fulfilled or to personally inconsequential needs.
- Motivate people by appealing to their higher-level needs (i.e., their turn-ons). Don't give them painkillers, which appeal to their lower level leads and temporarily remove dissatisfaction but do not really motivate (Frederick Herzberg). To help managers apply these basic insights, as part of our management training, we teach them to use a 35-item questionnaire found in the appendix of *Managing for Excellence, A Guide to Developing High Performance in Contemporary Organization* (John Wiley, 1984) with the employees who report directly to them. The instructions for this survey direct leaders to ask their employees to answer each item twice. The first time, they are to circle a number from 1 to 5 (1 being "very little" and 5 being "great extent.") The second time, they are asked to put a square around the number that describes how they would like to be. We teach managers how to develop personalized motivation strategies for individual employees on items within which there is the great span between high squares (how employees would like their bosses to be) and low squares (where there bosses are now).
- Make sure all forms and expressions of approval are commensurate with a level and quality of performance (equity theory). Our major checkpoints here are the corporate staff's review of all performance evaluations and promotion recommendations.

- Deliver on your promises and don't promise anything you can't deliver (expectancy theory). We explicitly instruct all of our managers to be precise, accurate, and complete, especially during the hiring and promotion process on all expectations for an employee's new work. Employees have more than adequate channels to complain about false or empty promises, and we monitor compliance with this tenet at all of the exit interviews we do with employees leaving us.
- Make sure all desirable behaviors are followed by a pleasant consequence even if that be a simple thank you, and manage the consequences of performance (reinforcement theory). The things we do to make sure this principle is consistently applied hospital-wide are covered in detail in chapter 6.

KEEPING EVERYONE IN THE KNOW:
Weekly Division Meetings

One characteristic of quality institutions is that information flows freely and is shared generously and not hoarded by individuals as a method for exercising power over or against others. Employees who are called to high standards of work need as much information as possible about everything that directly or indirectly affects their work. Leaders serious about quality will share everything possible that may be of assistance in getting a top-notch job done. Paltry little cannot or should not be shared—personnel matters and strategic market initiatives that are competitive secrets before they are approved by the Board and ready for implementation by our management team, for example. Virtually everything else should be an open book to employees.

At our hospital, we have tried hard to communicate with our employees but truth be told we are not satisfied at the level of our effectiveness. Structural barriers present in all institutions account for some of our lack of success. Some information never reaches some people at all. As it makes its way through the institution, other information arrives in a distorted, piecemeal, and sometimes even contradictory renditions. Then, too, the accuracy and completeness of information is sometimes affected by the relative skill, thoroughness, and discernment of individual department heads and supervisors who serve as the organization's informational mediators.

The principal mechanisms we use to keep people accurately up to date on information pertinent to them on an ongoing basis are the hospital's regular weekly corporate staff meetings and regular divisional meetings. Every Monday morning from 8:00 AM to 10:00 AM and often beyond, the corporate staff meets to share what the CEO and each vice-president consider important information to be shared at specific levels of the organization. Within two days of these corporate staff meetings, each vice-president is expected to pass along this information to all of his or her department heads. They, in turn, are expected by week's end to pass the information to their supervisors and through them to rank-and-file employees. This week, I shared 35 items to be passed along through my division. These items included a report on our just completed board-corporate staff retreat, the addition of several new employed physicians, a contract proposal for emergency services, an update on CQI initiatives, recent developments related to our managed care strategy, new personnel announcements, and on-going marketing projects—plus much, much more.

There are times when especially significant and important information must be transmitted in a uniform and consistent way—for example, when we announced our intention to begin an open heart surgery program, when we proposed an alliance with two previous competitors, and when we explained the conditions under which the newly approved alliance was permitted to proceed. Consequently, during any typical year, there will be anywhere from four to six full management staff meetings conducted by the Hospital's CEO or chief operating officer. In addition, at least four times a year, the president holds open forums for all employees to ensure that especially vital information directly reaches them in a clear, undiluted, and consistent fashion.

Individual vice-presidents are strongly encouraged to meet with the employees in each of their departments at least three times a year. Employees, in turn, are constantly urged to raise questions of their department heads and vice-presidents whenever they have a concern or would like to verify the accuracy of some rumor. Managers, as well as employees, need to be in the know.

A month or so ago, our president and CEO, Don Creamer, held a public forum to announce the effective date of our alliance, the alliance's mission, value, and vision statements and the consolidation plan schedule set for the first 18 months. Employees asked questions about things like the consolidation implementation teams, about wage, benefits, and policy changes, about the elimination of positions and about the process to be applied in the identification and disposition of employees displaced by the consolidation of services.

Communication must be, as people are fond of saying, two-way. All of the meetings described above are structured as forums in which information is communicated from the rank and file up through mid-management, up to the corporate staff, as well as settings in which top-down information is shared. Department heads and supervisors are trained and evaluated on their effectiveness in ensuring two-way communication with their employees. In good organizations, bad news travels fast to the top. As Ron Zemke put it in *Total Quality* (July 1993), "Successful leaders get 'real-time feedback.'"

Our employee manual contains this important statement:

Employee Questions Concerns, and Complaints

The Williamsport Hospital & Medical Center is committed to providing all employees with opportunities to ask questions, express concerns, make suggestions, and register complaints. Every member of management, from supervisor to president, is committed to maintaining open two-way communication with the hospital's employees. Employees are encouraged to use the normal chain of command to express their concerns and complaints. In most cases the supervisor will be able to resolve the problem.

Employees have the right to respectfully discuss their concerns with any member of management, including supervisors, department heads, and corporate staff, without fear of reprisal or retaliation.

Managers who forbid their employees to use these approved channels or who threaten employees who use these channels with reprisals or recriminations will themselves be subject to disciplinary action, including the possibility of termination.

Employees who prefer to submit their concerns in writing or who wish to bring their concerns to the president's attention may use the IMPACT system. An employee who submits a signed IMPACT statement will receive an acknowledgement within five working days. All signed IMPACT submissions will be answered by the president or his designee.

When an employee's problem cannot be resolved satisfactorily through one of these avenues, he may use the hospital's grievance procedure.

We repeat the content of this statement incessantly: at orientation for new employees, at mandatory annual employee training programs, in management training, in our weekly newsletter and in all of our individual personal contacts with managers and employees.

The hospital regularly conducts organizational climate assessments. Individual employees have available to them the IMPACT statement process. IMPACT statements addressed to anyone on the corporate staff or on the management team may be dropped into a box in the cafeteria. Employees who do so are guaranteed a response within five working days. Our training programs strongly encourage all employees to have frequent informal contact with managers and employees participating in or affected by any of their work activities. Finally, accessibility and approachability are characteristics that we constantly look for and promote in all of our management team.

SEEING THE CUSTOMER FIRST HAND:
The Corporate Staff's Work-a-Day-in-My-Shoes

The story goes that one day someone asked Kevin White, the former mayor of Boston, why he stopped bringing people from Harvard School of Business to work in City Hall. "They know how to administer," he responded, "but they don't know the people in the neighborhoods." John Le Carre, the British spy storyteller, made essentially the same point when he said, "A desk is a dangerous place from which to watch the world." Quality and customer service calls for regular contact between customers and a company's executive leadership. Even those of us who acknowledge this basic tenet about executive leadership in a service setting acknowledge that we need to do far more to implement this principle and practice than we are currently doing.

At the hospital we have done some things for starters. We have purposely not created a position for a patient care representative or advocate or a CQI department. Such moves give the impression that customer service is one person's or one department's job, not everybody's. Managers and employees are personally responsible for identifying and resolving customer problems and meeting customer needs. Corporate staff officers personally follow up on all problems and complaints brought to their attention. A corporate officer personally visits the home of any one of the very rare number of people who indicate on a patient satisfaction form that he will not return to The Williamsport Hospital & Medical Center for services in the future. Corporate officers regularly visit patients throughout the hospital. But probably the most beneficial way that the executive staff at our hospital has stayed close to the customer is through our work-a-day program, the so-called work-a-day-in-my-shoes (see Resource 3-4).

Every month corporate staff officers are expected to spend one full day working in a different department in the hospital. Whenever possible, they are asked to *work*-a-day, not *walk*-a-day in someone else's shoes. It doesn't always quite work out that way but if it did,

---

Resource 3-4.   Work-a-Day Guidelines

1. All members of the corporate staff should participate.
2. Work-a-Days should be scheduled well in advance, for example, quarterly.
3. "Work-a-days" should include a well-rounded representation of clinical, service support, and ancillary departments.
4. Corporate officers should spend at least four uninterrupted hours—preferably the *entire* shift—on each work-a-day.
5. They should rotate to all days and all shifts.
6. Corporate officers should not simply observe, but if possible and practical actually participate with their mentor.
7. They should complete at least six—preferably 12—work-a-days a year.
8. Corporate officers should begin when their mentor or host begins and wear appropriate clothes.
9. They should decide in advance with their host or mentor the type of work-a-day they will have (for example, an hour with each of a number of employees or four to eight hours with one or two employees).
10. Get department heads providing support service to do work-a-days in their customer departments and department heads to do work-a-days in departments providing them with ancillary support services.

---

every department in the hospital could have one of our corporate staff working in their department at least once a month. Almost always, corporate staff officers work in a department for a day come back with at least one idea for improving customer services—not infrequently on a matter that has been suggested in the past but not truly appreciated until seen first hand. After one of Don Creamer's work-a-days, maintenance established a regular schedule for replacing ceiling tiles. Our COO, Steve Johnson, worked a day last year with our environmental services people. The result—a new regimen for reconditioning areas as they were cleaned. A corporate work-a-night led to a year-long CQI project to reduce noise at night on the nursing units. Over the course of the years, we have learned through experience that there are certain ways of maximizing the benefits from this regular practice.

The possibilities for expanding the frequency of management hands-on contact with the customer are limitless. Hospitals are 24-hours-a-day, 365-days-a-year operations, yet 99 percent of the time, the corporate and departmental levels of management are present on campus only during daytime working hours. Institutions aspiring to reach ever higher levels of quality service will institute practices that ensure an executive presence on every shift, on weekends, and on holidays. Second and most especially, third-shift employees often lack a sense of belonging and identification experienced by day-shift employees. Ideas like our 10-year old monthly C.A.R.E. pizza round for night-shift employees need to be multiplied to ensure regular contact between senior management and employees and to ensure that moments of truth transpire during the times of the day, week, and year when senior executives are typically not at work.

It can't be repeated often enough that most effective teaching and learning about quality is imitative. Employees tend to do what we do, not what we say and fail to do ourselves. Programs of the kind I am suggesting should not entered into lightly. They can easily become the gimmick of the month. Once begun, they must be maintained in the long run—forever and a day as a matter of fact—if employees are to continue to learn from the example of managers and to consistently imitate it themselves over time. Continued over the long hall, such practices can serve as the most eloquent manifestation of walking the talk that I can imagine.

79

THE CORPORATE DREAM: No Layoffs

There's a strong link between morale and quality service. Positive morale, we believe, ensures the delivery of quality and the achievement of quality ensures the maintenance of a positive morale. In the words of Blanchard and Spencer, "People who feel good about themselves produce good results, and people who produce good results feel good about themselves." Morale and quality are mutually reinforcing. The higher the morale, the better the quality of people's work; the better the quality of people's work, the higher the morale.

The literature on the aftermath of layoffs indicates that the opposite is also true: demoralized employees working in a company that downsizes through layoffs experience a reduction in productivity and in quality and become part of a drastic weakening of the company's culture. Surviving employees feel guilty, become insecure, and allow things to fall between the cracks. Survivors feel frustrated, angry, and betrayed because they think an implicit contract—the security of long-term employment in exchange for dogged loyalty—has been broken. Quality suffers because people become so worried about losing their jobs that they stop doing them.

No senior management team can or should ever promise that there will never be layoffs. Sometimes unpredictably urgent and drastic economic necessities leave no alternative. Japanese companies long committed to lifetime employment are now facing this jolting fact of life and will continue to do so at least through the mid 1990s. Still, it is surprising that even companies that see a connection between morale and quality and acknowledge that layoffs inevitably reduce morale and therefore make quality more difficult to obtain seldom articulate explicit goals and strategies to render the necessity of layoffs less likely. If high morale promotes quality service and layoffs foment poor morale, why don't more companies strive to maintain quality through strategies aimed at eliminating the need for layoffs? If quality is the competitive edge and layoffs blunt it, why do so many senior executives see the avoidance of layoffs as a humanitarian consideration rather than as a business requirement? Explicit planning to avoid layoffs is not only the right thing to do, it is the financially responsible thing to do. As Don Creamer often says, "It is possible to do well by doing good."

We have explained our philosophy about layoffs innumerable times to our employees over the last decade (see Resource 3-5). Don Creamer has publicly said that we cannot promise there will never be layoffs. He has promised that we will do everything that is institutionally responsible to avoid them. This contingent pledge, however, is not a promise of unconditional job security. When all else fails, we fire persistent nonperformers as a matter of regular practice—an average of 26 employees a year over the last 10 years. We promise to try not to lay off our good performers. We also promise *to fire* their opposites.

During the past 10 years under Don Creamer's leadership, the corporate staff has studiously and persistently endeavored to implement programs and policies that have enabled us to avoid layoffs. Some hospitals—for example, those with a financially undesirable payor mix or those run poorly for years—may find it hard if not impossible to avoid layoffs. These are some of the initiatives we think have helped us to avoid layoffs at least so far:

- We established an explicit no-layoff goal and an explicit, detailed plan that will increase the possibility of success.

Resource 3-5.   10 Business Reasons for Avoiding Layoffs

1. At the least, morale falters; it often plummets.
2. Customer service quality suffers—in the first dimension of quality (personal service) almost unquestionably and potentially in the second and third dimensions (system service and service outcomes).
3. The company's service culture is threatened.
4. Surviving employees feel guilty and are prone to more mistakes.
5. Relationships between managers and employees become strained.
6. Insecurity becomes rampant.
7. Employees feel betrayed.
8. The atmosphere rubs off on customers.
9. Layoffs can exacerbate the business climate of a community struggling to develop economically.
10. Union-organizing activities often begin.

- We developed a winning strategic plan that contains each of the elements described in quality rule 12 in chapter 1—high quality service must be preceded and supported by high quality strategic planning.
- We took steps to grow the business. A few of the many examples:
  —In 1985, we won a 10-year contract with the City of Williamsport to provide basic and advanced life support services for the city. One out of every three of our admissions is an emergency room patient and one out of every 10 emergency room patients is an admission.
  —Ten years ago, we avoided the convenient care center fad and developed strategically located family practice satellites with employed physicians. Today, most of the family practice offices in our community are operated by physicians who are hospital employees.
  —Seven years ago, we established a joint venture with more than 150 of the 200 physicians in our community.
  —Two years ago, we began an open heart program. We plan to be doing 400 cases in two years.
  —Four years ago, we reorganized the outreach and case management functions of our rehabilitation center. Admissions are up 60 percent. Outpatient volumes are up dramatically as well.
  —Five years ago, we expanded our occupational health program into a comprehensive effort that now has exclusive agreements with more than 100 businesses.
  —Four years ago, we initiated a sports medicine center that has exclusive agreements with every school district and college in the area.
- We have taken steps to reduce costs. (Over the years, our hospital's operating costs have run in the lower range of hospitals nationally.) For example:
  —Through planned attrition over 10 years we have reduced full-time equivalent employees from 1,346 to 1,175.
  —Through seven years of intensive CQI initiatives that emphasized value, we have saved substantially but not completely documented savings. (For example, we have saved over $4 million through our product procurement committee.)

—Through our participation in the Voluntary Hospitals of America Procurement Network, we have been purchasing all kinds of equipment and supplies and have received loans at rates much lower than those available to our competitors.

—We save $500,000 a year because we are self-funded for workers compensation and do not pay current workers' compensation rates.

In a favorite daydream of mine, I like to imagine the hospital's cafeteria wall filled with the names of the companies throughout the United States that have laid off employees during the 1990s. Next to this almost endless catalog and standing alone on the side I like to imagine the words, "The Williamsport Hospital & Medical Center: After twelve years, still no layoffs." That standard of employee relations, I firmly believe, will guarantee levels of quality service that has an incalculably higher dollar value than the cost of planning and achieving a corporate no-layoff dream.

4

Enabling People to Deliver
Quality Through Training

*Training defines the difference between hot air and
a genuine commitment to go-beyond quality.*

There's only one way to make quality improvement continuous—and that's through training. We often remind ourselves of the words of New Jersey's Senator Bill Bradley who once said: "When you're not practicing, remember, someone, somewhere is practicing and when you meet him, he will win." The objective of training is to spark our employees' drive and to develop the skills necessary to provide go-beyond quality during each moment of truth in a cycle of service in each of the three dimensions of quality: personal service, user-friendly systems, and healthcare outcomes and processes.

In determining what kind of training we needed for whom, the corporate staff asked three questions:

- What quality outcomes do we want to achieve?
- What institutional, managerial, behavioral, systems, and clinical capabilities do we need to develop to support our quality outcomes?
- What training designs for what participant targets do we need to deliver to develop and maintain these support capabilities?

We have already described and explained our quality outcomes. Briefly put, this is what we want to be the result of our service delivery:

Go-Beyond Quality Outcome—exceed customer expectations:

An enthusiastically positive objective customer experience and subjective customer perception during every key moment of truth in the service cycle in each of the three dimensions of quality against the following outcome criteria:
• C.A.R.E.: reliability, tangibles, assurance, responsiveness, and empathy.
• TQM/reengineering and MEDIMPROVE: efficacy, appropriateness, availability, timeliness, effectiveness, continuity, satisfaction, efficiency, respect and caring.

Next, the corporate staff determined the capabilities required to successfully achieve this quality outcome in a sustained way hospital-wide. To ensure the delivery of go-beyond quality in all three of these dimensions of quality, a hospital needs:

• *Managers effective in their role as employee team builders and leaders.* Assumption: Over the long run, employees treat customers the way they are treated, customers feel the way employees feel, and employees must *want* to do something before they can do it.
• *An interpersonally skilled and technically competent and motivated workforce.* Assumption: It is *people* who C.A.R.E., *people* who devise and activate smooth delivery systems, and *people* who practice medicine.
• *A specific plan by which moments of truth are pervasively transformed into magic moments in every department of the hospital.* Assumption: Effective teams need service blueprints or game plans and need to be trained in their execution.
• *A continually updated cadre of service managers.* Assumption: Department heads and supervisors must establish and monitor the attainment of service standards and ensure the continuation of magic moments and the correction of counter-encounters.
• *Managers with an in-depth knowledge of how to analyze and improve service systems.* Assumption: It is the job of managers to work with their people to devise hassle-free service systems, to get people to use them, and to fix or replace them when necessary.

- *CQI teams supported by CQI team leaders and facilitators.* Assumption: Teams do quality improvement better than isolated individuals, and teams guided toward efficient team processes and team results do quality best of all.
- *CQI tools specialists available to all teams when they are needed.* Assumption: CQI is a learned craft, not an intuitive art form. Teams need CQI tools expertise as a standby source of support.
- *Managers and employees skilled at bringing out the best in people and dealing with the worst in people.* Assumption: Success in interpersonal and managerial performance is as difficult, if not more difficult, than success at clinical work. Consequently, personal skills training should be as high a priority as clinical training.
- *Mechanisms through which fresh ideas and perspectives come from the outside on a regular basis.* Assumption: Customer-responsive organizations must be outside-in-organizations driven not only by market research but also by state-of-the-art research.
- *A clinically and technically superior medical staff and clinical support managers and professional personnel.* Assumption: Healthcare knowledge and skills quickly become obsolete and must be incessantly deepened and updated.

Having decided what quality meant to us and what capabilities we needed to increase our chances of making our quality mission a mission accomplished, we designed our CQI training plan.

HOW TO TREAT EMPLOYEES AND CUSTOMERS: The Managerial Leadership Course

Our success in delivering go-beyond quality depends on the competence of our managers more than on anything else. Through training, managers develop the will and the ability to motivate, inspire, and enable their employees to consistently deliver on the three dimensions of quality. Managers learn how to:

- Discern the most urgent and important high-priority needs of all of their customers during key moments of truth.

- Organize, deploy, monitor, and evaluate the delivery of services in response to these identified needs.
- Understand the current and future business and healthcare environments in which we must compete.
- Initiate new approaches and techniques to help us succeed in increasingly complex and ambiguous times.

In Peter Drucker's sense of these terms, managers become better at marketing (identifying customer expectations and requirements) and innovation (responding in creative ways to the needs identified). Since *Harvard Business Review* the late 1980s, it has been fashionable to disparagingly contrast leaders and managers. According to this model, the job of leaders is to involve themselves in lofty, extra-mundane, high-level activities that ensure that the right things are done. Once given the step-by-step recipe book by leaders, managers are then engaged to follow the leader's instruction in getting the already dictated right thing done in the right way.

So, at the same time CQI gurus espouse empowerment for rank-and-file employees (power to the people) as an ultimate unquestioned and supreme CQI value, managers who are responsible for their employees' quality performance and their customers' experience of satisfaction have been disenfranchised and relegated to the role of functionaries. This way of thinking about things is misguided and counterproductive.

Managers *are* leaders. Managers are leaders in a business or organizational setting. Just as employees are empowered within the bounds of common sense and judgment to do whatever necessary to move heaven and earth in satisfying the customer, so managers ought to be empowered within the bounds of common sense and judgment to discern the right thing to do as well as to make sure it is done in the right way. The empowerment of managers confers upon them the role of leader.

Our radiology department is a busy place. Most of our patients are unscheduled and for a community of our size, the department does a whopping number of tests—80,000 a year. Some years ago, despite the great staff we had working there, the systems in place led to long delays for our patients within radiology, delays for patient tests in other departments, and long physician waits for test results. Our patient satisfaction rating was 82 percent. Under the leadership of our front office supervisor, Denise Clark, the service systems were revamped. Denise and her staff adjusted staffing schedules, redesigned the space, planned and monitored renovations, selected a more efficient computer system, and began and continued intense service training—the works. The result: patient satisfaction ratings are now 95 percent positive. We are grateful to have department heads and supervisors like Denise throughout the hospital.

No one above the immediate supervisory level can determine in detail what is right in every aspect of hands-on service delivery. We need people like Denise to help us make those judgments. CQI driven organizations consider their managers and supervisors to be leaders— not mindless Pavlovian administrators—and treat them as such. As James M. Kouzes and Barry Z. Posner put it in *Credibility* (Jossey Bass, 1993): "Enlightened managers know that serving and supporting unleashes more energy, talent, and commitment than commanding and controlling."

As we have seen, total quality management requires the management of two relationships: the relationship between management or supervisors and employees and the relationship between employees and customers. The effective management of the first relationship is a prerequisite for the effective management of the second relationship. Our managerial leadership course is designed to teach managers and supervisors to make their relationships with employees productive and amicable. CQI is of necessity a team effort. The basic supervisory leadership course is aimed at qualifying every manager as an excellent team builder and leader.

The managerial leadership course (see Resource 4-1) is all about getting our managers to treat our employees like gold and to motivate, enable, and empower them to treat our patients like gold. In this course, they learn to manage the task and relational dimensions of their work. In a word, they learn the behaviors that will make them effective managers. An effective manager is one who creates an environment in which employees do whatever is needed to deliver the best results for the customer in ways that help the hospital achieve its quality goals and the employees fulfill their personal and professional aspirations.

The staff in our laboratory would do anything for their department head, Tom Schnars. Three months ago, after Tom had been the department

---

Resource 4-1. The Managerial Leadership Course

1. Managing the Pepsi Generation: The TWH&MC's Managerial Expectations   The ways in which the healthcare environment and modern workers have changed requires hospital managers to change in 10 basic ways.

2. You're Hired: Getting the Best Candidate for the Right Job   It's easier to hire the right person than to train the wrong person. Hospital managers are expected to learn and implement the behavioral model of interviewing, which is based on the assumption that the best predictor of future behavior is past behavior.

3. How Am I Doing? Measurable Performance Evaluations—1   The most important evaluative function of a manager is to give regular, ongoing verbal feedback to employees on their performance. Participants learn how to give effective positive verbal reinforcement and constructive criticism.

4. How Am I Doing? Measurable Performance Evaluations—2   The annual performance evaluation is a summary, not a surprise; an exchange of information, not a report card; a forum for positive feedback and an event designed to improve future performance. Managers are taught how to prepare, conduct, and document employee performance.

5. It Takes One Rotten Apple: Dealing With the Problem Employee   Participants learn how to identify problem employees and how to use progressive discipline to change their behavior or, when that proves impossible, to change the employee.

6. Time Management—1   Participants identify their own personal work-related time-wasters.

7. Time Management—2   Participants select time-management techniques to eliminate their time-waster and to bring more of their boss- and system-imposed time under their own personal control.

8. Turn-Ons and Turn-Offs   Participants learn the principal theories of motivation: content theories (Maslow, Herzberg, ERG Theory); Process theories (Equity & Expectancy Theories), and Behavioral Reinforcement Theory. They then apply these theories by selecting from 30 practical ways to motivate people.

Resource 4-1. The Managerial Leadership Course
(continued)

---

9. What Kind of Boss Am I: Status and Authority Aren't Enough Managers learn the eight tasks of leadership, a flexible model for selecting the appropriate management style (The Situational Model of Leadership), and the prerequisites of successful managerial performance.

10. United We Stand: Teamwork Participants learn the importance of and need for teamwork in institutions and how to and how not to build and sustain teamwork.

11-13. The Williamsport Hospital & Medical Center's Administrative and Personnel Policy Manual Participants learn the hospitalwide policies of The Williamsport Hospital & Medical Center.

14. Project Planning and Management—1 Participants learn how to set goals and objectives, checkpoints, and time frames and how to manage individuals, teams, and project schedules.

15. Project Planning and Management—2 Managers learn how to promote group cohesiveness and enthusiasm, how to keep members informed, and how to promote creativity and perseverance.

16-20. CQI Basic Tool Training CQI team members learn the basic tools used in implementing quality improvement projects.

---

head of our laboratory services for only about a half a year, all of the staff in the laboratory nominated him as C.A.R.E. Employee of the Month. Anyone you ask in the laboratory would tell you that they don't squander accolades lightly. When our folks in the laboratory say you're good, you are *good*. Tom is a personal model of customer service without compare, and he's as responsive to his staff as he is to our patients. I guess that's why the corporate staff received a petition signed by all of the laboratory staff last week requesting that whatever other organizational changes we planned to make, Tom would remain their department head.

Leaders are responsible for results. The basic leadership course teaches our managers the organizational quality goals they are responsible for achieving. Managers learn the hospital's mission, value, and goals and ways that they can effectively achieve these institutional ideals in a dramatically transformed and reformed healthcare environment with a dramatically different post-Pepsi generation of employees. Managers learn all the basics of management, including:

- Negotiating individual and group objectives and expectations that are derivative of the hospital's corporate goals. For example, in accordance with corporate goal 1—Customer Service, environmental service staff were trained as roving ambassadors of C.A.R.E. In our last patient survey, 95 percent of our patients said that our environmental service staff members were *always* courteous. Five percent said they were *usually* courteous.
- Monitoring, coaching, and facilitating employee performance toward the achievement of these goals. For example, in support of corporate goal *4* (Support and collaborate with members of our medical staff), nurse managers for years have worked with our nursing staff to accommodate the reasonable preferred ways of our physicians.
- Managing the consequences of employee and group performance by reinforcing successes and by constructively correcting false starts and missteps. For example, in compliance with corporate goal 6 (Implement a seamless delivery system), our corporate staff regularly gives feedback to managers whose efforts must be coordinated to attain go-beyond quality: nursing and discharge planning; admissions, emergency room, environmental services, and nursing; nursing and dietary; nursing and pharmacy; human resources and operations.

The relationship that has the greatest effect on employee productivity and morale is the relationship between employees and their immediate supervisors. Our department heads and supervisors are responsible for creating the kind of relationship with their employees that leads employees to have a sense of accomplishment, of worth, and of self-respect and a desire to serve. If managers fail to create this kind of environment, however generously strewn, seeds of CQI will fall on barren soil.

QUALITY C.A.R.E. BOOSTERS:
Maintaining Healthy Employee Behavior

Several months ago, I traveled to Memphis, Tennessee, to speak to the managers of the Baptist Memorial Healthcare System. I got to the front desk of the Adam's Mark Hotel at 11:56 p.m. I hadn't eaten all day and was famished. So I asked the clerk if I could get something to eat. He politely apologized and explained that room service closed at midnight. The porter who had brought me from the airport, went behind the counter, pulled out a menu, opened it, and gave it to me, "What would you like, Mr. Mannello?" I said, "Anything. I'd settle for a chicken sandwich." Twenty minutes later, having reopened a kitchen that had to be closing for the day, he appeared at my door with a beautifully presented full-course hot chicken dinner! Whenever I think of the Adam's Mark Hotel, I will think of that go-beyond gentleman. When he recalls the tip I gave him, I'd like to hope that he might occasionally think of me. Getting people other than those who are naturally disposed to the heroic to perform like this porter demands training—lots and lots of training.

Like any perishable product, training programs have a limited shelf life. We believe that is as true of the basic quality C.A.R.E. course given to the board, corporate, and management staff and all of the employees 10 years ago as it is of any other training program. Training programs need to be conducted on a regular basis to keep quality ideals and goals fresh in everyone's minds, to motivate employees to continue their efforts toward go-beyond quality, and to reemphasize the meaning, the purpose, and the methods of ensuring favorable customer outcomes in the three dimensions of quality. That's where our annual quality C.A.R.E. boosters come in.

Every year we take all of our employees through a mandatory one-and-a-half to two-and-a-half hour session intended to provide them with the motivation and the skills they need to participate in an active way in making a thousand things one percent better every day. Last year our course was entitled: "The What, The Why, and The How of Continuous Quality Improvement." This year, our program has a title "Quality C.A.R.E. in Trying Times: The Scoop," a session devoted to the federal, state, and local trends transforming the healthcare environment, the implications of these trends on our corporate strategies,

93

service operations, and financial prospects, and the plans we formed to work with our employees, our physicians, and our volunteers to thrive in an era of managed competition.

The purpose of this session was to maintain the high level of employee morale required to ensure go-beyond quality at a time when federal and state reform initiatives, pressures from all sides to reduce costs, headlines about layoffs elsewhere, and the prospects of an alliance with our former competitors were causing widespread employee concerns and anxiety. Presented in a popularized and illustration-packed version, the major points covered in the session were these:

- *What—the trends—healthcare costs too much:*
  —Our two largest customer payors—business and government consider their healthcare to be too expensive or non-affordable.
  —American businesses complain that healthcare is the one principal cost of doing business that makes it hard to compete internationally.
  —If healthcare cost increases were to continue at the rate of growth experienced in the last 10 years, the federal deficit would explode to unmanageable proportions.
  —Efforts at all levels and in every sector abound to bring healthcare cost increases to the level of general inflation.
  —Some external pressures will force us to reduce costs; we will have to initiate other cost-reduction efforts ourselves.

- *So what—the impact:* Without proactive change, these pressures could negatively alter our financial stability:
  —Before reimbursement by Diagnostic Related Groups: There was a time when it was almost hard to lose money.
  —After reimbursement by Diagnostic Related Groups: The guarantee of financial viability disappeared.
  —The era of managed care: Welcome to the capitalist world of the free market where there will be winners *and* losers.
  —We've got to continue to develop services and programs that the community needs, especially those that are at least break-even and for which people currently need to leave the community to get.
  —We've got to concentrate on value—that is, quality improvements that improve efficiency.

94

—Sixty-percent of our costs are labor related; 60 percent of our cost-cutting measures need to be labor related.

—Our goal in effecting these efficiencies is to do so without layoffs. Here is our plan.

* *Now what—what a class-act group does in uncertain times:*

  —C. *Courtesy*: specific behaviors.

  —A. *Attentiveness*: specific behaviors.

  —R. *Responsiveness*: specific behaviors.

  —E. *Empathy*: specific behaviors.

The result of the training: after a year in which dental and vision coverage as well as Christmas turkeys and hams were eliminated, and 156 employees had their hours reduced from 40 hours a week to 37.5 hours a week, our employee organizational climate assessment hit all-time positive ratings.

Human resources staff members designed this program, and they run as many sessions of these courses and run them at whatever times necessary to get the entire workforce through our program each year. Last year, the program was run 85 times at different hours in the morning and afternoon of the work day, at 7:00 PM, 9:00 PM, 1:30 AM, and 2:30 AM in the morning to accommodate second and third shifts. This year, we will be able to reach all of the employees in 50 to 75 sessions run during similar hours of the day and night. Class sizes typically range from 15 to 75 people, and on the off-shifts run as low as two to three employees. Barring an emergency that justifies cancellation, sessions are always run regardless of the number of employees who turn up to participate in them. In this way, each and every employee comes to understand that we are very serious about our quality values and that each of them plays an indispensable part in helping us become all that we can be.

One potential topic for next year's quality C.A.R.E. session is using TQM tools. The object of this session will be to teach all employees the underlying rationale and scientific methodology involved in applying total quality management tools to the improvement of service delivery systems in language that everyone can understand. It will be an attempt to put into popularized basic and simple form the tool training long delivered for our managers, supervisors, and CQI team leaders and members. Based on the last chapter of Karl Albrecht's book, *The Only Thing That Matters* (Harper, 1992), the topics that will be covered during this two-hour session will be selected from among the following tools:

- The moment of truth chart.
- The cycle of service chart.
- The service blueprint.
- The why-why diagram.
- The how-how diagram.
- The tracking chart.

Vice-presidents, department heads, and supervisors are expected to make it possible for all of their employees to attend even when their participation requires supervisors to back-fill, pay overtime, or bring on extra help. The cost of participation at our hospital is not thought of as an expenditure with no payback but as an investment in our ability to deliver a level of quality that translates into financial success well beyond the cost of paying employees to attend and others to fill in. Our average hourly rate is about $12 an hour. We have about 1,500 employees. The time employees spend in this training would cost $25,000. We only back-fill for about 10 percent to 20 percent of participants. Let's say additional labor costs amount to $5,000. Since we use no consultants, and design and deliver this training ourselves, this training costs us about $3.30 per employee per year. We consider this cost peanuts when contrasted with the results. The management staff of our hospital is so convinced that training is necessary to ensure the success of our quality efforts that discussions about the costs of making it possible for everyone to attend are seldom if ever broached. Ongoing regular quality C.A.R.E. training has become as much a matter of daily routine as breakfast, lunch, and dinner.

NUTS AND BOLTS I: Managing the Moments of Truth

The Little League center fielder was having a rough day. The first two batters lofted fly balls in his direction. The youngster dropped them both. In frustration he threw down his glove and kicked it. The third batter followed with a sky-high fly ball to center field. It came down and hit him right on the head. He stomped off the field into the dugout, walked up to the manager, and said, "You just can't catch a ball on this baseball field."

Many service executives and managers say the same sort of thing about delivering world-class quality in their organizations.

Exceeding customers' expectations for each of the dimensions of quality—personal service, user-friendly systems, and healthcare outcomes—by transforming every moment of truth in the cycle of service into a magic moment is a neat idea, isn't it? But how do you even try to make that happen everywhere for everyone at all times? The course, "Nuts and Bolts I: Managing the Moments of Truth," was designed to make the go-beyond quality dream an everyday customer experience in each and every one of the hospital's departments. (Resource 4-A in the Appendix outlines this course.)

At the end of the course, all of our participants, our corporate staff, our department heads, and our supervisors were charged with developing a departmental-quality service plan, a plan that delineated the following in minute detail:

- Each department's customers.
- Their moments of truth (contact points during which they made judgment points about the quality of our service).
- Their precise expectations during each moment of truth.
- An explicit description of who, what, when, and how high-priority customer expectations would be surpassed by our actual service delivery.

About 180 department heads, supervisors, and rank-and-file employees participated in the development of the hospital's quality service plan some six years ago. We required every department to submit a quality service plan and honored those submitting the best as part of our first annual Chairman's Quality Award Program. Every year, departments are required to submit an update of their existing quality service plan and a description of how they will train employees to practice what we promise we will do.

If an organization believed that its success was assured by conscientiously executing a strategic plan based on quality as the competitive advantage, its management team would never worry that a competitor could read and thoroughly understand the details of their plan. Knowledge, contrary to Aristotle's cerebral view, is not virtue. Knowing the right thing to do is no guarantee that one will do what is right. Quality institutions execute the transparently simple. Impostors manipulate customer perceptions to come across as the genuine thing. Quality organizations are win doctors; carbon copies are spin doctors.

NUTS AND BOLTS II: The Fine Points

It's hard for an organization to stay committed to quality over the long haul, as it is for many of us married folks who stay together for better or worse—but not for long. What's the secret? Someone once told me: "I don't know whether I pray because I believe in God or whether I believe in God because I pray." I believe that our actions need not be determined by our attitudes and emotions but that our actions shape and reshape our attitudes and emotions. It may seem a huge stretch, but I think the same thing can be said of quality. Organizations don't hang in there on their original commitment to quality when the going gets rough because their belief in quality is unshakable. Rather they remain faithful to their quality ideals because they keep finding creative ways of expressing and practicing them. Nuts and Bolts II (Resource 4-B in the Appendix) is an example of what I mean.

What The Williamsport Hospital & Medical Center did in Nuts and Bolts II: The fine points are not so important as the utility of how we did it. We took Karl Albrecht's book, *At America's Service* (Dow Jones-Irwin, 1988), and came up with a simple way of exposing our entire management staff to ideas that built upon the basic ones espoused there. The book has 15 chapters. So, we came up with the idea of the 15-15-15 club. What that came down to was, the corporate staff agreed to spend 15 minutes on 15 separate occasions to summarize the essential points of each of the 15 chapters of the book at the corporate staff's weekly Monday morning meeting. Vice-presidents then were asked to get their department heads to do the same thing at their weekly divisional meetings. Consequently, at the end of about four months, the corporate staff and department heads were exposed to and discussed additional ideas that would help them implement the basic ideas they and their management staff had mastered from Albrecht's book, *At America's Service.* The book didn't necessarily have to be *At America's Service,* though my bias is to say, that was not a bad selection.

Here's the process:

- Carefully select a book whose content you have determined will be most helpful in promoting managerial initiatives to support quality.
- Get your corporate staff to spend less than a half hour discussing the insights of this especially insightful book.
- Duplicate that process at the department head level.
- Articulate the expectation that what corporate staff members and department heads have learned will be shared and put into effect by the people who have hands-on responsibility toward your patients and other customers.

It's a marvelous way of doing things. Everyone is required to pitch in. Therefore, everyone is inclined to buy into its execution and success. Whatever else is going on, this ongoing kind of activity takes just a little time and would contribute mightily to anyone's quality effort and provide a freshly invigorating injection of creativity into what can be a dogged and repetitive effort to sustain the achievement of an organization's quality aspirations and commitment.

CLOSING THE SERVICE GAPS:
Making Sure Nothing Falls Between the Cracks

In the basic leadership supervisory course, we give our managers and supervisors the know-how to manage their relationships with their employees in ways that will make it possible for them to manage the relationships of our employees with our customers. Through Nuts and Bolts I and II, we give our entire management staff the wherewithal to methodically identify their most important customers, their high-priority expectations during those most critical moments of truth so that we can as individuals, as members of a department and cross-departments, react in ways that genuinely surprise the people we are privileged to serve.

So what next? Things always seem to fall between the cracks. The most creative things that institutions are doing in the face of this reality is to promote collaboration, coordination and consolidation wherever any one or all three of the Cs result in a better experience for the customer. Now that staff from our satellite employed physician offices belong to our CQI teams, we have reduced the incidence of snafus between hospital staff and staff from our physician's office. A regular training offering of ours, Closing the Service Gaps (see Resource 4-C), moves the quality ball up field from the current scrimmage delivery line toward the goal line of go-beyond quality.

Closing the Service Gaps is built on the ready acknowledgement that there's a whole lot we can do to deliver services better. This course is based on *Delivering Quality Service: Balancing Customers Perceptions and Expectations,* by Valerie Zeithaml, A. Parasuraman, and Leonard L. Berry. The basic supervisory leadership course is intended to make all of our managers and supervisors effective employee team leaders, and Nuts and Bolts I and II are intended to help departmental teams set up responsive delivery systems. This course is intended to help managers, supervisors, and CQI team members eliminate any possible gap between the service as perceived by the customer and the service as expected by the customer.

Participants learn to identify and to close the four principal gaps that create customer dissatisfaction when perceived service and expected service do not coincide. These gaps are:

- The gap between customers' service expectations and management's perception of customers' expectations.
- The gap between management's accurate perception of customers' expectations and service delivery specifications or standards.
- The gap between service quality specifications and service delivery systems.
- The gap between service delivery and external communication to customers.

Put simply, the four gaps are: not really knowing what customers expect, having the wrong service quality standards, not translating the correct service quality standards into service systems that truly deliver on them, and making promises that don't match delivery.

During the first four sessions, our human resources staff teaches participants how to find and to remove the root causes of these four quality gaps and to manage the entire service delivery process so that customers receive and perceive that they have received go-beyond quality. In the fifth and six sessions, participants are given an overview of the principal CQI tools used in analyzing and improving the functioning of the hospital's service delivery systems. Principal sources for this last section of the course are selected ideas gleaned from W. Edwards Deming, Joseph Juran, and Philip Crosby. Like the basic supervisory leadership course and Nuts and Bolts I and II, this course is offered regularly to managers and employees involved in CQI efforts throughout the hospital.

FACILITATOR TRAINING:
Ensuring Group and Task Maintenance in CQI Team Meetings

The hospital's key resource as facilitator and facilitator trainer is our management engineer, Bob Ireland. Over the course of time, as CQI efforts have expanded, we have developed a need to clone Bob so as to have effective CQI facilitators available to all of our CQI teams. At the time of this writing, the hospital has just under 50 trained CQI facilitators and is planning to have a complement of about twice that size in one year.

We like to train our CQI facilitators in small groups—ideally made up of not more than six to eight people. Training sessions (see Resource 4-2) are designed to be participative and to provide opportunities for the application of the skills and tools that are taught. Participants learn the dynamics and stages of group formation and work, methods for keeping groups focused on the tasks and on sustaining group cohesiveness, and rules on whether and how to intervene to keep the group focused and productive. Participants also get an opportunity to understand the underlying scientific methodology involved in using TQM tools and get to practice the tools in what we like to call the basic CQI tool kit:

- Brainstorming.
- Multi-voting.
- Pareto charts.
- Gantt charts.
- Affinity diagrams.

Resource 4-2.   Facilitator Training

SESSION 1
This session addresses the team, team participant roles, team dynamics, facilitation skills, and team productivity.

Learning Objectives
Participants learn:
- The role of a facilitator.
- The role of team leader and team members.
- The stages of team development and the facilitator's role during those stages.
- How to coach and support team leaders.
- How to diagnose and intervene in group dynamics.
- How to resolve conflict and move stalled teams forward.
- How to make team meetings productive.

SESSION 2
During this and the following sessions participants work as a team on a CQI project practicing the use of various CQI tools. This is a workshop approach with participants assuming various roles as team members, leader, or facilitator.

Learning Objectives
Participants will learn to use the following tools:
- Brainstorming
- Multi-voting
- Pareto charts
- Gantt charts
- Affinity diagram
- Flowcharting
- Opportunity statements
- Cause-effect analysis

SESSION 3
During this session, participants continue to work as a team on their CQI project with an emphasis on data collection and conversion of data into information. This includes some very basic statistics.

Resource 4-2.   Facilitator Training *(continued)*

Learning Objectives
Participants learn to:
- Use check sheets, run charts, and control charts.
- Structure a simple customer survey for data collection.
- Convert observations data into charts and graphs.
- Calculate mean, median, standard deviation, and percentiles.

SESSION 4
During this session, participants develop a new process, select alternatives, develop an implementation plan, and establish monitoring systems.

Learning Objectives
Participants learn to:
- Use a prioritization matrix, process decision control charts, activity networks, and control charts.
- Structure a storyboard display.
- Recognize the key assets of quality function deployment for ensuring customer focus.

The goal is that upon completion of this training program participants will feel comfortable to assist CQI teams in keeping on focus, remaining productive, and using CQI tools.

- Flowcharting.
- Cause-effect diagram.
- Opportunity Statements.

Facilitator training at The Williamsport Hospital & Medical Center is provided on an as-needed basis to the CQI teams actively pursuing quality improvement at any given time. For example, when one of our interdepartmental teams broke down badly trying to collect information really pertinent to their problems, Bob helped the team develop the data collection forms and analytical procedures that moved their project forward. Bob has developed and is delivering advanced CQI tools training to the graduates of his basic course even as I write this chapter.

JUST-IN-TIME TRAINING (JITT):
CQI Tool Training When It Really Helps

A long-time ago when I was young enough to know everything, I actually tried to teach English to high-school seniors. It was a disaster. One day in the middle of my class, the school's principal walked by, peered in through a back window, and observed a boy in the back row reading the sport's page. After class, he informed me that he was going to call that student to his office and reprimand him for what he had done. "No," I pleaded with the principal, "please let him read the sport's page. He's probably the only person in the whole class who is learning anything." I used to give myself low grades for my failure with my disinterested students in those days. Now distanced from the unhappy ordeal by time, I am a little easier on myself because I believe that for whatever reason, the students were just not motivated or ready to learn.

Psychological readiness and timing are important aspects of any effective learning. We have found that our CQI team members master the CQI tools when they are at stages in their work that call for the actual use of those tools. They learn the tool best when they need the tool most. They quickly master it as they use it. As the Romans used to say: "*Faber fit fabricando*"—that is, a carpenter learns by carpentering. Our employees' successful use of CQI tools provides them with the gratification of seeing them actually work. Maybe the Chinese proverb says what we are trying to say best of all: "I hear and I forget. I see and I remember. I *do* and I understand."

We've used CQI team leadership and facilitation as two slightly differing functions. A facilitator's job is to manage the process through which teams do their work. The CQI's team leader's job is to lead the team toward solutions that are substantively responsive to service delivery deficiencies.

Successful teams are characterized by two attributes: they complete their job (task maintenance) and they are cohesive and collaborative (group maintenance). The role of team leaders is to make sure the team makes progress toward the substantive completion of its work. The leader's role is to get this group task done. The role of the facilitator is to make sure that as the task is being accomplished, all members are engaged and contributing. The facilitator's role is to see that when this task is done, the group is willing to work on future projects. Many times, one person plays both roles.

For example, the team leader of a CQI group working on reducing waiting times in a service area needs to make sure the proper data analysis, root cause identification, and improvement options are identified and that the best solution is selected and implemented. The team facilitator needs to be sure members are behaving in ways that facilitate task accomplishment (e.g., ask pertinent questions, offer pertinent information, resolve conflicts, summarize) and avoid behaviors that make the job harder to do (e.g., dominate the discussion, interrupt, argue, get off on tangents, offend others). We also see team facilitation and leadership as rotating functions—that is, functions that can be performed by any member of the team whose intervention or behavior results in advancing the work of the group and the process through which the group achieves its goals.

Our intention, therefore, is to provide facilitator and leadership training to as many of our managers, supervisors, and employees as we possibly can. In addition to conducting facilitator training on a more frequent basis, we are considering the inclusion of our four-session facilitator training program as a concluding module in our basic supervisory leadership course next year.

BRINGING OUT THE BEST IN PEOPLE:
How Employees Like to Be Treated

There is an unspoken sentiment in many hospitals that years of long, hard, and rigorous training are required to equip and qualify healthcare providers in performing medical procedures and managing healthcare regimens. At the same time, it is widely thought that the interpersonal dimension of quality care (personally dealing with customers and employees) comes naturally or not at all. It can't be taught. We hold a different view. I like to say that even I could become a world-renowned neurosurgeon—transplanting heads on Saturday morning in the emergency room on an outpatient basis with discounts for senior citizens. Certainly a lot easier than dealing with the varied, complex, unpredictable vagaries of human behavior . . .

Care providers need as much ongoing support and training in the interactional dimension of their jobs as they do in the technical dimensions. Consequently, in addition to our management and ongoing C.A.R.E. boosters, we try to provide different kinds of courses on dealing effectively with people.

One such course, which we run regularly, is a course based on the book *Bringing Out the Best in People: How to Enjoy Helping Others Excel,* by Alan Loy McGinnis (see Resource 4-3). In the course of this three-session seminar, we teach our managers and other interested employees McGinnis' 12 rules for bringing out the best in people. There are, of course, countless books like McGinnis' book that can serve as a foundation for continuing courses on interpersonal skills. For example, two excellent possible texts on which to build courses have been written in the past few years by Stephen Covey: *The Seven Habits of Successful Leaders* (Simon & Schuster, 1989) and *Principle-Center Leadership* (Simon & Schuster, 1992). Our human resources staff members are in the process of developing courses on these two texts right now.

DEALING WITH DIFFICULT PEOPLE:
When Customer (or Employee) Isn't Right

People are fond of saying that the customer is always right. Nonsense. The patient who, without provocation, spit in the face of one of our radiology technologists, was not right. We teach our managers and employees that although our customers are not always right, we want to be the very best in dealing with them when they are wrong.

Over the years, we have found Robert Bramson's book, *Coping With Difficult People* (Dell, 1981), to be a wonderful reference and guide in helping our caregivers deal with a wide assortment of different

---

Resource 4-3.   Bringing Out The Best in People*

SESSION 1
- Expect the best from people you lead.
- Make a thorough study of the other person's needs.
- Establish high standards for excellence.
- Create an environment in which failure is not fatal.

SESSION 2:
- If they are going anywhere near where you want to go, climb on other people's bandwagons.
- Employ models to encourage success.
- Recognize and applaud achievement.
- Employ a mixture of positive and negative reinforcement.

SESSION 3:
- Appeal sparingly to the competitive urge.
- Place a premium on collaboration.
- Build into the group an allowance for storms.
- Take steps to keep your own motivation high.

*Based on: *Bringing Out the Best in People: How to Enjoy Helping Others Excell,* Alan Loy McGinnis.

---

people they confront in their daily work. Bramson emphasizes that although we can all be difficult at times, only a small percentage of people are habitually difficult. These habitual offenders actually prefer their troublesome style of acting because it works for them. His main point is that we perpetuate their difficult behavior by our typical responses to it. So, throughout his book, he teaches concrete specific alternative methods of dealing with the most typical kinds of difficult people we are likely meet.

In our eight-session course (see Resource 4-4), we teach our employees to deal with hostile-aggressives: the Sherman tanks, the snipers, the

Resource 4-4.   Dealing with Difficult People

Sample Session
Hostile Aggressives at a Glance

WHAT THEY DO	WHAT THEY DO TO US	WHAT TO DO TO THEM
SHERMAN TANKS		
1. Overwhelm you	1. Confusion	1. Stand up for yourself
2. Attack you	2. Put out of commission	2. Give them time to run down
3. Run over you	3. Fight—rage	3. Jump in
4. Overpower you	4. Flight—cry or flee	4. Carefully get their attention
5. Pulverize you	5. Inability to cope with the situation	5. Get them to sit down
		6. Speak from your own point of view
		7. Avoid fighting
		8. Be ready to be friendly
SNIPERS		
1. Take pot shots	1. Reduce to inaction	1. Surface the attack
2. Wound you	2. Leave no apparent options • ignore or confront? • their way, look silly	2. Give sniper choice besides fighting
3. Shoot from behind the cover of social conventions and humor	3. Get sniped at the longer problem remains	3. Check out group's opinion
4. Often snipe over long unresolved problems	4. Vicious cycle set-up	4. Deal with problem
		5. Take preventive measures
		6. Don't handle someone else's problems
		7. Intervene on your own behalf

Resource 4-4. Dealing with Difficult People *(continued)*		
WHAT THEY DO	**WHAT THEY DO TO US**	**WHAT TO DO TO THEM**
EXPLODERS		
1. Throw tantrums	1. Take us by surprise	1. Give them time to run down
2. Go out of control	2. Bewilder us	2. If they don't intervene
3. Blow up unpredictably	3. Sometimes provoke us to anger	3. Show that you take them seriously
4. After the flare-up —typically blame and suspect others	4. Make us too emotional to want to understand by reducing us to silence, passivity, or a tantrum of our own.	4. Get some privacy with them or a breather from them
		5. Get them to sit down
		6. Speak from your own point of view
		7. Avoid fighting
		8. Be ready to be friendly

exploders. We teach them also how to deal with the rest of the trouble-some characters in Bramson's gallery of interpersonal horrors:

• The Compleat (sic) Complainer—people who think that all of the problems they experience are caused by external sources: for example, "Alibi Ike" problem employees who cannot perceive much less acknowledge their shortcomings or the rare but real patient who is impossible to please.

• The silent unresponsive person—for example, patients who begrudgingly and minimally answer questions about their physical history but withhold pertinent information that has not been requested.

• Super-agreeables and other wonderfully nice people—for example, employees or patients who cannot abide friction and have real problems but to do not mention them.

• The negativist—for example, the occasional employee who doesn't make the effort to win attention through constructive problem-solving but does so by perpetual problem-finding.

- Bulldozers and balloons: The know-it-all experts.
- Indecisive stallers.

For each of the categories of difficult people, Bramson provides insightful instruction into:

- What makes them tick, where they are coming from, how they got to be the way they are.
- What they do, how they act, what their tell-tale behaviors are.
- How we typically respond to their unbalancing and obstructive behavior and thereby cause a repetition of it.
- What we should do specifically instead of what we normally do to make the exchange productive and to get on with our business.

At the end of the course, participants come to understand times when they themselves act like difficult people and leave with detailed concrete strategies for handling the occasional difficult person who may crop up in their work and in their lives away from work.

Management Development Program

In her book, *Celebrating Italy,* Carol Field writes that the people of a remote mountain town called Villa Santa Maria in Abruzzo refer to their town as *"Il Paese dei Cuochi,"* the village of cooks. Villa Santa Maria continues to send "phalanxes of its residents" across the world as chefs in restaurants, great hotels, and embassies. Because he had eaten food in Rome cooked by chefs from Villa Santa Maria, Field Marshall Kesserling purposely spared the town when the Germans bombed Abruzzo during World War II. Quality does not go unnoticed.

Like the townsfolk of Villa Santa Maria, we at The Williamsport Hospital & Medical Center have a bias for doing it ourselves. We are strong believers in letting the doers do the design and the planning as well as the implementation. We have a deep, but largely unspoken aversion to consultants. We like to see those who are free with advice stay around and witness the effects of their counsel and to clean up the mess when unanticipated consequences result from an implementation of their wisdom.

On the other hand, we can become inbred and parochial and thus regularly need the perspective of others outside of the hospital to expand our thinking and to identify long-cherished paradigms that no longer work. We try to make the words of an anonymous poet our own way to keeping our collective minds open:

> I kept six honest serving men.
> They taught me all I knew.
> Their names were What and Why
> And When and How and Where and Who.

To ensure the insertion of fresh ideas and perspective, we have had a management development and supervisory development program conducted by external presenters for years. Our management development team is made up of department heads. They plan and administer three to four half-day or whole-day sessions off campus for the management team each year. Members of the management development team select the topics, speakers, the agenda, and run it from dollars allocated for this purpose entirely themselves.

Over the years, we have had programs on the following kinds of topics:

- Motivating employees.
- Installing a new computer system.
- The phases of change and the skills for successful adaptation to change.
- Paradigms.
- Union prevention.
- Stress management.
- Healthcare trends (3 different programs).
- CQI tools.
- Team building.
- The psychology of change.
- Managed care.
- Improving quality and reducing costs: Two complementary ideas.
- The post-patriot generation: What makes today's workers tick.

- Conflict management.
- The needs of organizations, the needs of employees: making them one and the same.

Several years ago in response to an expressed desire on the part of our supervisors to have similar training programs, we instituted a supervisory development team that does for their peers what the management development team does for department heads and management staff.

Just recently, our management development committee has looked back on 10 years experience in conducting these kinds of programs and has developed a list of suggestions and guidelines for bringing them off successfully:

- The management development committee should be a multidisciplinary committee of eight to twelve members with adequate representation from nursing.
- The committee should have a representative from the corporate staff.
- The committee should sponsor three programs a year (more than that is hard to bring off.)
- Programs should be timely and relevant and should focus on the managerial, technical, and team-building needs of the group.
- The corporate staff member should participate in topic selection but not dominate or impose topics.
- Off-site seminars are more effective than programs held on campus.
- The safest way to pick a presenter is to select speakers heard by and recommended by at least one member of the committee. (The size of the required fee is no guarantee of presenter quality.)
- Half-day programs are more popular and effective than full-day programs.
- Committee members should delegate details of the set-up to others:
  —Room set-up is crucial.
  —Room temperature must be right.
  —Personally check out room prior to seminar.
  —Have really good meals!
  —Have a social aspect to each meeting (summer picnic in afternoon for example).
- Provide a simple questionnaire to evaluate all aspects of the program.

HOSPITAL-SUPPORTED CLINICAL STANDARDS AND TRAINING: A Good Bedside Manner Isn't Enough

Our customers' most important expectation is, of course, a favorable medical or healthcare outcome. Meeting that expectation requires a highly trained medical staff and professional clinical support team. We are blessed to have both in spades—to a startlingly exceptional degree for a town of 35,000 people and a service area with about 150,000 people. Our physicians and nurses, for example, recently scored in the superior range when compared to their colleagues in the over 800 hospitals that make up the Voluntary Hospitals of America (VHA-argued by some to represent the very best community hospitals in the country.) Typical of the clinical support we have throughout the hospital, our rehab professionals (physical, occupational, recreation, psychological, and speech therapists) exceed regional and national rates reported by the Functional Improvement Measurement System for rehab inpatients and do so in substantially shorter lengths of stay. (I could go on and on—I'm so proud of our people—but I'll spare you.)

The point is, yesterday's successes don't guarantee tomorrow's results. We consider all of our staff to be professionals—everyone, including our dietary, maintenance, and environmental service employees—because we think of *all* of our employees as people who support favorable medical outcomes. Consequently, we put strong emphasis on practice standards and decentralized training across the board for our medical staff, for our clinical staff, and for all our other professional support personnel—and that's everyone! (Resource 4-5 shows an overview of The Williamsport Hospital and Medical Center's training programs.) Here are but a few examples of how we support our MED-IMPROVE efforts:

Medical staff credentialing and training

According to our hospital's bylaws, all physicians seeking initial appointment to the staff have to be board certified, or be an active candidate seeking board certification, by the specialty board relevant to the physician's area of practice or department in which privileges are requested. The term active candidate is defined as a physician who has

Resource 4-5.   Training at-a-Glance at
The Williamsport Hospital & Medical Center

Quality Outcome	Required Capability	Training Response at The Williamsport Hospital & Medical Center	Participants	Frequency and Length
An enthusiastically positive objective customer experience and subjective customer perception during each key moment of truth in the service cycle in each of the three dimensions of quality against the following outcome criteria: • C.A.R.E.: reliability tangibles, assurance, responsiveness and empathy • TQM/Reengineering • MEDIMPROVE: efficacy, appropriateness, availability, timeliness, effectiveness, continuity, satisfaction, efficiency, respect and caring	Effective managerial team leaders	The Managerial Leadership Course	All department heads and supervisors—mandatory	18 sessions 1-2 times a year
	Motivated, interpersonally skilled workforce	Quality C.A.R.E. Basic and Booster Course	All employees—mandatory	Orientation and 1 time a year afterwards
	Managers who can develop and update service plans	Nuts and Bolts I	All department heads and supervisors—mandatory	6 sessions 1 time a year
	Trained service managers	Nuts and Bolts II	Department heads—voluntary	1 time every 2-3 years
	Managers trained in system analysis-improvement	Closing the Service Gaps	Department heads and supervisors—mandatory	1 time a year
	Facilitator tool training	Basic and Advanced Facilitator Training	Selected leaders—voluntary	Ongoing

114

Resource 4-5.   Training at-a-Glance at
The Williamsport Hospital & Medical Center *(continued)*

Quality Outcome	Required Capability	Training Response at The Williamsport Hospital & Medical Center	Participants	Frequency and Length
	Available tools specialists	Just-In-Time-Training	CQI Team Members	Ongoing
	Interpersonally advanced staff	Bringing Out the Best in People Dealing with Difficult People	All employees—voluntary	1 time each a year
	Outside-In Management Staff	Management Development Program	Management Staff	3-4 times a year
	Medically/ Clinically/ Technically Standards and Training	Hospital supported technical standards and training	All employees—decentralized	Ongoing

graduated from an accredited residency in that specialty within five years prior to the date of making application for staff membership. In addition, the hospital sponsors a generous continuing education program for its employed physicians—about half the physicians in our area—and opens up all of our family practice lectures to all members of our medical staff.

Continuing education in nursing— the clinical ladder

The Williamsport Hospital & Medical Center has had a nursing clinical ladder for seven years. Requirements for each of the steps in the ladder are:

- Clinical Nurse I—Minimum of 10 Continuing Education Points (CEPs) annually; attends mandatory CPR, fire training, patient carries, and infection control inservices.
- Clinical Nurse II—Minimum of 15 CEPs annually; attends mandatory CPR, fire training, patient carries, and infection control inservices; maintains intravenous certification.
- Clinical Nurse III—Minimum of 25 CEPs annually; attends mandatory CPR, fire training, patient carries, and infection control inservices; maintains intravenous certification.
- Clinical Nurse IV—Minimum of 35 CEPs annually; attends mandatory CPR, fire training, patient carries, and infection control inservices; maintains intravenous certification; maintains certification as a CPR instructor.

Training in support departments

All of our nonclinical, support departments have formal training programs on the technical aspects of their work. The training program in our environmental service department is typical:

- Orientation—Each new employee receives three full days of training one-on-one with a supervisor.
- Flexible OJT—Each employee receives on-the-job training with a senior environmental service employee for whatever time is needed to bring the employee up to department standards.

- Post 90-day training—After an employee's first 90 days of work, one-on-one supervisory retraining may occur if necessary.
- Routine training—*All* employees receive reinforcement and updating training every six months.

Ken Blanchard points out that when you hire a new employee, you confront several possibilities: You can hire someone perfect (you the reader and I know that no one except the two of us falls into this category); you can hire someone who is trainable; or you can pray! The behavioral model of employee selection and our employee certification program are aimed at reducing our need for prayer. Once employees are certified, training is one of the few remaining human interventions available to make CQI work before we get down on our knees to ask for assistance from a higher power.

It is often said that there are three things that are important about real estate: location, location, location. Similarly, there are three things that are important about writing: rewriting, rewriting, and rewriting. There are also three things that are important for the continuous success of continuous quality improvement: training, training, training. CQI walkers train. CQI talkers don't. By their flip charts, you will know them!

5

Nurturing Self-Managing Teams and Empowered Employees

No one of us is smarter than all of us.

Two preschoolers were fighting over the rights to a little wagon. There was enough room for both, but each wanted to ride up front. Finally, after a lot of pushing and shoving, one of the tikes said: "You know, one of us could have a lot of fun, if *you* would get off!" Childhood habits die hard, and teams fail to produce extraordinary results because, like children, members refuse to subordinate personal objectives and agendas to a common vision and set of goals.

Given our tradition of rugged individualism, we Americans came to the factories ill-prepared for the teamwork necessary to make world-class products and deliver first-rate services. We failed to make the most of our resources, our advantages, and our capabilities because we fail to put it all together, together.

Now Americans are learning about teamwork with a vengeance. And so are we at The Willamsport Hospital & Medical Center. To prepare our staff for their CQI team efforts, we teach them the characteristics of superior teamwork developed by NASA during our managerial leadership course:

- Mutually set team goals.
- Understanding and commitment to team goals.
- Clearly defined, non overlapping member roles.

- Atmosphere that encourages development.
- Decisions based on facts, not emotions or personalities.
- Efficient task-oriented meetings that focus on improvement.
- Discussions that involve all members.
- Members listening to and showing respect for each other.
- Problem-solving versus blaming.
- Frequent performance feedback.
- Informed members.
- Pride and spirit.
- Free expression of feelings and ideas.
- Cooperation and support of members.
- Tolerance for conflict with emphasis on resolution.

These are the ideals that all of our CQI teams strive to emulate. These characteristics are the charter by which our self-managing teams manage their CQI work.

Customer-Focused Cycle of Service Teams

We've had seven cycle of service teams in place for about four years now. These cycle of service teams are the groups within which all of the good things we have to say about CQI converge and get put into practice (see Resource 5-1 for our cycle of service team guidelines). These teams concentrate on our customers and on their highest-priority needs. They scrutinize all of the key moments of truth of our typical customer categories during the entire cycle of service. Team membership is interdepartmental and multidisciplinary. These teams operate continuously, and their rotation of members ensures continuity. They possess all of the ingredients of the ideal CQI team model.

Each of these cycle of service teams devotes its time and efforts to one of our most typical customer categories:

- Elective admission patients.
- Same-day surgery patients.
- Outpatients.
- Emergency room patients.

Resource 5-1. Guidelines for Cycle of Service Teams

Each cycle of service team is assigned a specific segment of the patient population served at The Williamsport Hospital & Medical Center. The responsibilities of each team are to understand the cycle of service a patient experiences, monitor the care and services provided during that cycle, identify and prioritize opportunities to improve care or services, and to initiate improvement projects or establish spin-off CQI teams to address the opportunity.

Guidelines for Cycle of Service Teams:

- Teams should define the cycle of service their patient population experiences and monitor periodically to identify any changes.

- Teams should review care and services with a critical eye at least quarterly to identify changes in performance or development of new quality variations.

- Teams shall report every six months to the operations committee or corporate staff.

- Teams should prioritize opportunities for improvement based on high-volume, high-cost, high-risk, problem-prone, or customer-sensitive needs.

- All CQI projects and spin-off teams must be approved by the MEDIMPROVE committee.

- Team membership must be expanded to include representatives from the areas involved in a CQI project.

- Each team should have a trained CQI facilitator.

- Teams should begin by defining the mission and goals of the project; this may be summarized in an opportunity statement.

- Each team should establish an appropriate timeline or Gantt Chart for the CQI project and monitor its progress.

- Team members should communicate team activities and progress to the managers and staff in their work areas to obtain input, keep them informed, and get buy-in.

Resource 5-1. Guidelines for Cycle of Service Teams
(continued)

- As solutions are implemented, quality standards and monitors of quality must be incorporated to ensure improvement occurs and is maintained.
- As a project is completed, a written summary report must be completed and submitted to the MEDIMPROVE committee for documentation.

- Cancer patients.
- Open heart patients.
- Patients of our satellite physician offices.

The targets of opportunity that the teams define may be a response to a deficiency in any of the three dimensions of quality (C.A.R.E., TQM, or MEDIMPROVE) at any point in the cycle of service. Each of the teams includes a variety of specialists from the departments through which patients travel as they progress along the cycle of service. For example:

Emergency Quality Team
Chaplaincy Services
Environmental Services
Emergency Services (R.N. and M.D.)
Radiology Services
Laboratory Services
Paramedic Services

Same Day Surgery Quality Team
Radiology Services
Physician Office Practices
Same Day Surgery
Heart & Lung Center
Gastroenterology
Surgical Services
Preadmission Testing

Elective Inpatient Quality Team
Social Services
Distribution Services
Dietary Services
Nursing Services
Rehabilitation Center
Laboratory Services
Utilization Review

Four years ago, when these groups were first established, the corporate quality council determined the membership of each group. In the course of a six-session training course, CQI team members learned their mandate, their function, and objectives and acquired the teamwork and CQI tools training needed to do their work. At a lunch hosted by other members of our corporate quality council, Don Creamer thanked the more than 70 team members for their work and spelled out the charter under which they were to operate:

- Team members were to elect their own team leaders.
- Each team was to work with its designated customer group and with departments through which their customer traveled in the course of their cycle of service to identify improvement opportunities consistent with the highest-priority customer needs.
- Teams were to present their improvement targets for review to ensure that they were responsive to the target customer's very highest needs or expectations.
- Team members were to update the quality council on a quarterly basis.
- Members were to develop other guidelines for team operation.

Once the teams were established and operating, the quality council delegated steering and coordinative responsibility for the cycle of service CQI teams to the MEDIMPROVE committee. The corporate quality council directed the MEDIMPROVE committee to establish guidelines for: activating cycle of service CQI initiatives; facilitating, coaching, motivating, and monitoring team activities; and reinforcing positive team activities and results through different kinds of visibility and expressions of appreciation.

Before any CQI project can go forward, the MEDIMPROVE committee determines whether or not the target of opportunity is: a key moment of truth in the service cycle (first dimension of quality: C.A.R.E.); a quality-critical process (second dimension of quality: TQM); or a high-cost, high-volume, problem-prone healthcare concern (the third dimension of quality: MEDIMPROVE). Once they get started, team members get opportunities to report on their progress and their successes to the corporate quality council and the MEDIMPROVE committee and receive various forms of recognition and rewards. But more about that later. Resource 5-2 shows some of the projects our CQI teams finished this year.

Departmental CQI Teams

Organizations are a kind of living body made up of discrete organs or parts. In a hospital, we call these parts departments. For a hospital to really deliver for its patients, these parts or departments have to work together. That is why, even though departments are distinct from one another, we have been trying to impress upon them that they are not separate. Consequently, over the course of the last five years, we have encouraged our so-called departmental CQI teams to function as members of interdepartmental teams and to focus on customer priorities that bridge the gaps across departments. (Resource 5-3 shows our guidelines for departmental CQI teams.)

Our five-year-old Chairman's Quality Award Program described in chapter 6 provides the mechanism through which a manageable number of doable, high-impact quality-improvement projects are received on at least an annual basis from each and every department throughout the hospital. I'm amazed at how frequently I'm asked something like this at speaking engagements: "What if some department heads don't buy into this quality stuff?" My answer: "Around our place, there's an alternative—they would get an immediate opportunity to buy into some unemployment stuff." Quality is not a departmental option. It is a formal explicit job requirement. Department heads get evaluated on quality. They get rewarded and promoted on quality. It rarely becomes necessary to do anything punitive to managers who do not buy into quality because the kind of managers we have would consider that selling out.

Resource 5-2. Hospitalwide Cycle of Service Teams: CQI Project Synopsis

CQI TEAM	PROBLEMS	ACTIONS	OUTCOMES
Same Day Service	—Unsatisfactory preparation for exams —Patient delays because of scheduling problems —Availability of patient	—Specific actions taken to ensure completed charts —New guidelines to eliminate time-consuming, unnecessary steps in patient preparation	—Faster test results —More complete charts —Measurements being taken
Cancer Services	—Lack of physician consistency in admission for chemotherapy treatment —Tumor registry data collection	—Data collected, sent to MEDIMPROVE team —Site-by-site review of treatment data collected —Physician familiar with site will assist in setting up criteria for site —Cancer committee approval for collection of data established for each site	—Clinical pathway being formulated, with physician input. —Still in process

Resource 5-2.   Hospitalwide Cycle of Service Teams: CQI Project Synopsis *(continued)*

CQI TEAM	PROBLEMS	ACTIONS	OUTCOMES
Emergency Room	—Long admission times —No back-up system to support high-volume periods	—Multidisciplinary focus to streamline process with E.D. staff, attending physicians and admitting floors —Adequate staff to handle high-volume periods	• Faster admissions • Prompt service
Emergency Outpatient Testing	—Long testing delays —No updates to patients in treatment booths	—Faster testing turnaround time —informed patients	• Less waiting time • Improved customer satisfaction
Inpatient Elective	Services to Amish patients: —No insurance —Poor communication —Unique needs —Transportation/distance	—Provide discounts in return for cash payment —Meet on their turf —Provide consistent contact person here at hospital —No charge for television —Provide Hospitality Inn	• Increase in volumes • Satisfied customers • Cost-effective for both hospital and patient • Healthier population

Resource 5-2. Hospitalwide Cycle of Service Teams: CQI Project Synopsis *(continued)*

CQI TEAM	PROBLEMS	ACTIONS	OUTCOMES
Outpatient	Registration: —Accuracy —Wait times —Consistency Billing: —Lack of understanding by patient —Incoming calls going to all areas of the hospital	—Retraining of all clerks —Regular ongoing registration updates —Reduce registration screen —Error feedback to managers —Updated billing letter/readability index lowered —Installed 800 number for out-of-town patients —Revised all billing forms to achieve consistency	• Patient surveys indicated improvement in wait times (less than 5 minutes) • ICD-9 coding improvements • Registration clerks more knowledgeable thus reducing error rates • Calls to ancillary areas reduced to about 0 • Letter more easily understood • Billing form terms consistent with UB92 standardized form
Cardiac Surgery	—PAT for cardiac surgery patients takes 4 hours	—Trained volunteers with previous open heart experience and those who are in our CHAMPS program to escort our open heart patients through the PAT process —Decentralized the education of our patients	• PAT process has decreased by 60 minutes • Ongoing monitoring of the PAT process • Developed an informal questionnaire to highlight topics not covered in the hospital's patient satisfaction survey

127

Resource 5-3.   Guidelines for Department CQI Teams

Department CQI teams should be used as a management method to solve problems and improve care and services. CQI teams should also be used to develop quality processes and prevent errors.

Guidelines:

- Department CQI teams should consist of employees directly involved with the process being addressed.

- CQI team projects involving only issues and processes internal to the department should be approved by the department head and vice-president.

- Projects that involve processes interacting with others outside the department should be approved by the MEDIMPROVE committee and include representatives from involved areas and departments and a trained facilitator.

- CQI projects should be prioritized based on high-volume, high-cost, high-risk, problem-prone, or customer-sensitive needs.

- Department CQI teams should make communication of team activities to the entire department high priority and seek input and feedback frequently.

- At the onset of a project, the mission, objectives, opportunity statement, and schedule should be defined.

- All customers and customer needs involved in the process should be identified.

- Team emphasis should be on identifying and eliminating causes for quality variation.

- Upon completion of a project a summary report must be sent to the quality assurance department and a file maintained for documentation.

MEDIMPROVE CQI Teams

Gracious personal service and well-organized, smoothly run operations get a business so far but do not take it all the way to the quality target. People not only expect to have a good experience when they come for a service. They also expect to find a solution to the problem for which they sought out the service in the first place. Just the-way-you-like-it personal service and every time, on-time hassle-free service systems will get you into the ballpark and allow you to step up to the plate. But only solutions will enable you to knock the quality ball out of the park for your customers. For a hospital, that means delivering positive healthcare outcomes through the managed execution of best medical practices in the third dimension of quality—MEDIMPROVE. For us, zero defects *is* the uncompromising standard and measure of success in this dimension of quality.

In the jargon of the quality trade, The Williamsport Hospital & Medical Center has enviable input boosting the probability that our clinical process transformations will culminate in favorable, superior medical outcomes. In layman's terms, we've got a lot going for us to deliver on and surpass our patients' healthcare expectations. As we've seen, our medical staff, nurses, and clinicians have received superior ratings by external, independent evaluators. We have a generous, well-targeted capital equipment plan that makes us as high-tech as we are high-touch. For example, though we are a 300-bed hospital in a city of 35,000 people, we have had a magnetic resonance imaging service for six years, the most up-to-date heart catherization lab and cancer linear accelerator available, and have been providing lithotripsy and arthroscopy and laparoscopy services since that technology came on the market. Because of our family practice residency program, we enjoy a lively learning environment created by a superb faculty, a matched resident student body (our first picks typically pick us!), and a medical and clinical staff that participate in teaching residents and in learning beside them at our regularly scheduled physician lecture programs.

It is within this supportive atmosphere that our MEDIMPROVE CQI teams work under the coordinative aegis of our MEDIMPROVE committee. MEDIMPROVE CQI groups always include physicians (usually three or four), clinicians and other employees whose involvement is required to guarantee that completed living patient-management guidelines—always open to improvement—are indeed best practices. A team headed by our two employed infection control physician specialists—yes, The Williamsport Hospital & Medical Center has two of them (one, Dr. Gary Lattimer who played a key role in identifying Legionnaire's disease)—has developed infection control guidelines that have resulted in extremely low rates of all kinds of infections throughout the hospital. So far, MEDIMPROVE CQI teams have completed patient-management guidelines for patients requiring total hip or total knee replacements, coronary artery bypass grafts, preadmission testing for elective surgery, and outpatient laboratory testing. Currently, nine MEDIMPROVE CQI teams, all with heavy physician participation, are developing patient management guidelines for the following diagnoses or procedures:

- Congestive heart failure.
- Inpatient chemotherapy.
- Mastectomy.
- Cholecystectomy.
- Major small and large bowel surgery.
- Appendectomy.
- Angioplasty.
- Normal childbirth without complications.

The MEDIMPROVE committee is now working with our medical staff to develop a five-year plan for future work by MEDIMPROVE CQI teams. (see Resources 5-A and 5-B) These teams will either develop patient-management guidelines from scratch and put them into final form after testing them against externally developed guidelines or will begin with a patient-management guideline designed elsewhere and fine-tune, adapt, and otherwise improve the model to fit the circumstances of our setting.

The criteria against which we gauge the success of these patient-management guidelines are:

- Patient outcomes better than predicted rates.
- Consistent and efficient use of resources.

- Time savings.
- Cost savings.
- Improved integration of the continuum of care.
- Strong negotiating position for managed care contracting.
- Improved health status of community.

We also use Joint Commission on the Accreditation of Healthcare Organizations (JCAHO) criteria and make sure that as we do whatever is necessary to exceed the expectations of our customers and the professional standards of our caregivers. We are at the same time responding as completely as possible to JCAHO requirements. For example, our infection rates continue to run far below the average rates measured by the Communicable Disease Control Agency.

	Communicable Disease Control Agency Average	Versus	TWH&MC
Surgical Infection Rate	5%		1.3%
Non-Specific Infection Rate	5%		2.4%
Respiratory Infection Rate	7–41%		3.0%
Central Line Infection Rate	10–25%		2.5%

CQI SWAT Teams

Last night, I was making a batch of bread dough. The recipe called for six cups of flour. I accidentally put in 5 lbs.—roughly 12 cups. I also mistakenly used 2 tablespoons of yeast instead of one and five cups of warm water instead of a little less than three cups. Since I made three big mistakes instead of one small one, the bread turned out terrific.

Well, that's kind of what happened to us when we first starting using CQI SWAT teams about nine years ago. Our motto seemed to have been that old Lutheran dictum *"Pecca Fortiter,"* "Sin Boldly"— the by-word of all overly self-confident, fledgling cooks. To put it mildly, we made our share of goofs. We created a perfect model of how not to do it.

Here's what we did. We had a department with serious and urgent customer and employee problems. It was our emergency room. We put a SWAT team together. All of the members of the team were members of the corporate staff—yep, a CQI teams of six vice-presidents! The team planned the study—okay, the invasion. We explained our purpose, our methods, and how in the end, what we would do would be good for everybody. We interviewed all the employees in the department. We surveyed our physicians and our customers. We identified all the problems. We developed all kinds of solutions. We put in all new managers! We developed an implementation plan. The new managers put the plans into effect. Employee morale and customer satisfaction improved dramatically. What a success!

Buoyed by the results, we were ready to go on to the other departments. We asked for volunteers. Inexplicably, department heads and supervisors manifested no interest. In fact, they didn't seem to be around much when corporate officers were present. At one point, I thought they all went on vacation—simultaneously and perpetually! I swear I thought one of our department heads had died! Something was wrong. The obvious became clear—even to the six of us on the SWAT Team. We had spooked the management staff into paranoia. Surely, there was a more collegial, less-threatening, and more palatable and C.A.R.E.ing way of doing CQI—that is, if we did not want CQI to stand for Countless *Quisling Inspections*. We went back to the drawing boards.

We all knew better. People tend to support what they help create. Someone is not likely to put his foot through the bottom of a boat in which he was riding. So, future SWAT efforts were more self-evaluative. SWAT teams included the managers and staff of the service being studied as well as outsiders (*Nemo judex in causa sua*—that is, no one should be the sole judge in a case that affects him.) The insight about participation afforded by this simple remedy made subsequent efforts less adversarial and in the long run more effective.

As you may have surmised from this example, a SWAT CQI Team is a quality improvement team made up of "outsiders" and "insiders" to devise quick service solutions to serious, urgent service deficiencies within a department or among departments.

Since that time, SWAT teams have worked with our billing department, our rehabilitation department (which reports to me), our admissions department, our pre-admission testing department, and our laboratory department—with less disruption, far better cooperation and collaboration and highly positive results. The idea of SWAT teams remains invaluable. Sometimes, granted as a matter of exception, urgent service problems require immediate attention and quick solutions. When such circumstances arise, SWAT teams can be of enormous help if they follow the guidelines given in Resource 5-4.

Spin-Off CQI Teams

Ever since I began reading, speaking, and teaching about quality years ago, I've become a veritable value vigilante—a quality fanatic. Like saints, quality fanatics are much praised at a distance, but intolerable to live or work with.

About six months ago, I made my way to a supermarket in which the clerks remind me of Tom Peters' apt phrase: "TDC—thinly disguised contempt." Except that their contempt is not disguised, even thinly. It was raining. The store was busy. There were shopping carts all over the parking lot. A teenage boy dressed in a supermarket apron sat huddled in a outside corner watching the vehicles slalom around the carts. "Hey there," I called to the youngster, "do you work here or are you a volunteer?" He proudly responded that he was an employee. "Then get off your duff," I told him, "and earn your pay." I knew he was a nice kid when instead of giving me the expected middle finger, he got up to round up the carts. But 20 minutes later when I left the store, there he was again sitting watching the vehicular mayhem. I glared at him. He quickly jumped up and announced: "I'm movin', I'm movin'."

Two months later I was doing a work-a-day-in-my-shoes with one of our dieticians. She was emphasizing that tray delivery was a critical moment of truth and that she wanted to start a CQI team with a new tray deliverer as a member to develop a training program for this high-turnover position. As we approached the room where our new employee was delivering a patient's tray, he came out and faced me. I was now in a conservative suit with a vest. He put his face in his hands and muttered: "Oh, Lord, no!" It was my supermarket buddy.

Resource 5-4.   Guidelines for CQI SWAT Teams

1. Involve front-line caregivers as team members and information sources.

2. Emphasize the positive purpose of the CQI effort: to improve patient service and to create a better working environment—not to punish anyone for past failures.

3. Obtain commitment from team members to devote the time needed over the short term on what are quick-fix projects.

4. Clarify that the emphasis is on establishing appropriate quality through rapid implementation of corrective actions.

5. Use research data, rather than only personal anecdotal information, to identify service gaps.

6. Develop scientifically sound research instruments to gather customer and employee information, which will serve as the basis for decisions and recommendations.

7. Establish close monitoring for quality with assigned responsible individuals to fine-tune recommended actions as problems occur rather than plan out every contingency prior to implementation.

8. Include appropriate administrative representation so that team decisions can be made and actions taken without a delaying approval process.

9. Use the recommendations of the quality audit as a blueprint or departmental plan for the function in question.

10. Emphasize the prompt implementation of corrective actions.

11. Have the department head or management team make periodic progress reports on their quality improvements to the quality council.

12. Recognize, reward, and celebrate the improvements.

13. Keep monitoring the key quality indicators over time to watch for changes or trends.

14. Consider longer-term CQI team efforts after the processes are established with a view toward optimizing the use of resources and exceeding customer expectations.

Since then, a dietician, a staff nurse, a psychologist, and guess who, have developed an interactive video-training program for our dietary hosts. Dietary hosts are usually part-time employees who are students. The video training guarantees that all the new faces have the same old special touch. For years, delivering trays to patients used to be an improvised and perfunctory task with absolutely no quality controls. Today, it's a detailed, choreographed, and monitored encounter. For example, our hosts know how to properly identify patients without invading their physical or personal privacy, how to assist a patient who needs help without making them feel like a child (part of the training is based on Transactional Analysis!). Our patient surveys are telling us that the way they are served meals is almost as important as what they are served. Spin-off teams have developed from work-a-days, from cycle of service projects, and from departmental CQI efforts.

We take care to make sure that Spin-off CQI teams are not overly ambitious, respond to high-priority needs, and are properly supported. With these safeguards in place, spin-off teams provide the opportunity for ever-increasing numbers of employees to get directly involved in the business of quality. Three examples of Spin-off CQI teams from cycle of service teams are our occupational health team, Surgery/anesthesia process team, and outpatient registration team. (Resource 5-5 shows our guidelines for spin-off teams.)

Resource 5-5.   Guidelines for Spin-off CQI Teams

- All spin-off teams must be approved by the MEDIMPROVE committee.
- Spin-off teams should have at least one representative from the cycle of service team they originated from.
- Spin-off teams should have a facilitator.
- Spin-off teams must follow the same guidelines for CQI projects as the cycle of service teams.

Employee Empowerment Licenses

Everybody ought to be allowed one off-the-wall pet peeve. Here's mine: discussing ambivalent terms without defining them. In the current healthcare debate, we ask whether there is or is not a healthcare crisis without asking for whom, for how many, of what kind, and of what magnitude. And in discussions about quality, the rage is to go on and on and on like the EverReady rabbit about empowerment. Just empower everybody, whatever that means, and quality miraculously will break out all over.

For some, empowerment means telling employees they now have permission to do whatever they deem necessary to please the customer—no matter what. So some businesses just give employees the okay. Others add skills and the resources to the permission. They say, "You not only have the green light. We'll make sure you have the wherewithal to use your service license." Such employees all allowed and enabled to do their best by the customer as they see it. What is not often spelled out—the heart of the matter—are two questions employees still have. What are the limits of empowerment, and why should employees want to be empowered?

At The Williamsport Hospital & Medical Center, the limits within which all empowerment is conferred on individuals are set by a single general charge, two general rules, and five corporate goals that embody the hospital's mission and value.

- *General charge:*   Move Heaven and earth to exceed the customer's expectations.
- *Two general rules* (from Karl Albrecht's *Code of Quality*):
  —Think, use your common sense when ordinary procedures are not enough.
  —*Within reason,* bend the rules when necessary.

For example, a guest in our hospitality suite (free hotel accommodations on campus for out-of-town family members of our patients) called one of our operators for a morning wake-up call. Her response: "Certainly, Mr. Smith, what time would you like to be awakened?" After she hung up, a new operator said to her, "What does he think we are, a hotel?" The first operator told me that she responded, "You better believe we are, and we'd better find out what we're supposed to say if he calls back and asks for breakfast in bed!"

- *Five corporate goals:*
  —Treat our customers like gold (go-beyond quality).
  —Treat employees like gold (culture).
  —Increase market share (purpose).
  —Maintain competitive pricing (quality/price or value).
  —Partner with physicians (the new we).

In addition to these guidelines, the limits within which empowerment is conferred on all of our self-managing teams include two other directives:

- The corporate quality council must approve any proposed quality-improvement project of a high-priority customer requirement of the first magnitude.
- CQI teams must keep the quality council informed of their progress and success.

In chapter 6 when we discuss the indispensable part people play in the delivery of quality services, we will pay detailed attention to the other critical ingredient of empowerment—motivation. Why, after all, even when employees may and can, should they want to deliver go-beyond quality.

THE CQI RESOURCE LAB:
Where People Are at Home to Do Quality

After a recent talk in which I described our CQI resource lab, a participant told me that the few CQI teams they had in her very large hospital had to meet in a locker room. "Our CEO isn't into quality," she sheepishly and feebly tried to explain. Isn't into quality! I thought. I wonder what he *is* into? Miserable moments? Disastrous service systems? Record rates of morbidity and mortality? Patient dissatisfaction? Can you believe it? Sadly, that wasn't the first time I had heard that complaint.

People working on quality should not be reduced to the ranks of the institutionally homeless in our places of business. There is a deep connection between having a place of one's own and having a sense that what you do and who you are important. This connection is true of the thousands of literally homeless people on our city streets. It is true of people like Israelis and Palestinians. On a less global scale, it is also true of organizational groups that are constantly reminded of their meager influence and low status by not having a place they can call their own. Businesses give time, money, and space to the activities they consider important.

Our CQI lab is located in prime space, along our executive corridor leading to our employee cafeteria. It's highly visible. You've got to pass the lab whenever you're going to eat. The room is 16 feet by 16 feet and contains the following equipment, furniture and CQI aids, which we consider CQI lab needs:

- Table and seating for 6 to 14 people.
- Two-flipcharts.
- Very large whiteboard and markers.
- bulletin board or storyboard wall (10 ft. wide by 6 ft. high).
- computer and printer with software for:
  —word processing.
  —database analysis.
  —spreadsheets.
  —graphs and charts.
  —flowcharting.
  —CQI tools and applications.
- Quality-improvement reference literature and library:
  —Quality journals.
  —Reference texts.
  —Standards manuals (i.e., JCAHO, Nursing).
  —Dictionary and thesaurus.
- Television and VCR, video storage, and videotapes.

It is also nice to have:

- Storyboard area.
- Storage rack for flipcharts.

- Polaroid camera—to take pictures of whiteboard to transcribe later rather than having to copy before erasing.
- Desk with notepads, stapler, tape, and Post-it-notes.
- Space for each team to store materials.

All of our CQI teams—cycle of service teams, departmental CQI teams, SWAT teams and spin-off teams—use the resources of our CQI lab. We also make frequent use of the lab and its equipment and supplies when we conduct facilitator and CQI tools training. The CQI lab fosters quality-improvement activity—and quality-improvement results. That's why The Williamsport Hospital & Medical Center has a CQI resource lab. And that's why the CQI resource lab cannot be used by anyone except those working on a quality-improvement project. At all other times, it is kept under lock and key. As is the case in most hospitals, meeting-room space is at a premium at The Williamsport Hospital & Medical Center. Designating our most desirable real estate as the quality place was an eloquent reminder that quality is here to stay and that quality efforts provide the value to make this investment worthwhile.

THE WEEKLY CORPORATE STAFF CQI BRIEFING:
What We're Doing Really Means Something

The famous work of Elton Mayo at the Western Electric Plant in Hawthorne, Illinois, identified a remarkable connection between the human aspects of organizational life and worker productivity and quality. Mayo concluded from his studies that the most significant factor affecting the quality and amount of work completed by employees is to be found in the relationships among workers and their managers and other authority figures. He found that the attention his researchers lavished on the workers elicited feelings of self-respect, pride, and accomplishment and promoted synergistic teamwork and a strong sense of group affiliation. "The deepest human emotion," philosopher William James tells us, "is the craving to be appreciated." Unlike purely physiological needs, this psychological need is never satisfied. There is a limit on the number of steaks or the sundaes we can eat, but there's no limit on our pleasure in being noticed and appreciated. The most effective leaders are those who satisfy the psychological needs of their followers.

Remember the last scene in Arthur Miller's Play, *Death of a Salesman* where Willy Loman's friend Charlie says: "Willy was a salesman. He's a man way out there in the blue riding on a smile and a shoeshine. And when they start not smiling back—that's an earthquake." I have often thought that Charlie's words should be etched on the desk top of every manager.

Our corporate quality council tries hard to notice. The council receives regular briefings from CQI SWAT teams, cycle of service teams, and departmental CQI teams. The council reviews the work of our CQI teams not merely as a method for ensuring their continuation but because their work is so indispensably important that it *will be implemented.* One of the great pleasures of being a corporate staff officer is to sit in on these briefings. To see the remarkable patient service results the teams accomplish; to observe the enthusiasm and sincerity of employees dedicated as servants to their patients; to revel in the pride of the presenters who seem tickled pink to be associated with a class effort that yields first-class results. On several occasions, after a particularly competent and spirited presentation, I've said to myself: "Boy, I wish I had that on videotape. Nobody would believe it wasn't staged." Sometimes, I'm inclined to think that these briefings do more to increase the motivation of the corporate staff than they do to increase the motivation of our quality CQI team members.

NO GROUP IS A PARISH:
Destroying Departmental Parochialism

In *Preparing for the Twenty-First Century* (Random House, 1993), Paul Kennedy observes that there are three times as many independent, sovereign countries today than existed before the breakout of World War II. All of them have borders, armies, currencies, and narrow self-interests. This centrifugal shattering is spreading at a time when, from an economic perspective we were a global market, potentially a single all-embracing unit of economic activity. And things ain't much better locally or organizationally for that matter. Here too, people don't work and get along together all that well either. In too many organizations, individual departments judge their successes on intermediate products or contributive service rather than on the customer's complete overall satisfaction.

"The recall was on the fuel filter pipes, not on the electrical system. We're doing a great job!" a divisional chief at an automobile plant bragged after a recent expensive nationwide recall. Among other car manufacturers, Chrysler is trying to reverse this institutional isolationism by making teams of divisional managers jointly accountable for a car's total performance. At The Williamsport Hospital & Medical Center we have been working hard to create that same mind set: none of us succeed unless the overall service experience of our customer is superior. We promote this collegial attitude in three ways:

- Corporate modeling: For example, corporate staff members, like every other employee, are expected to acknowledge, smile at, and greet every one they meet on campus, hold doors open for others, pick up paper from floors, straighten up visiting areas that need it, and practice the leadership pledge with those who report to them.
- Managerial performance expectations and evaluations with interdepartmental cooperation as an explicit job expectation: For example, an otherwise technically competent and managerially exemplary department head was given a less-than-acceptable performance rating because he or she insisted on practices that adversely affected access and quality to patients in an interrelated department.
- The promotion, recognition, and reward of collaborative, departmental CQI initiatives: For example, one of the criteria in our annual Chairman's Quality Award Program explicitly encourages the submission of interdepartmental CQI proposals and projects.

Our corporate staff is a pretty tight group of professionals. Without question, we have our conflicts and squabbles. But seldom, if ever, does anyone outside the group see anything but a united front and a single position once a decision is made. We like to joke that we are a one-man one-vote group and that Don Creamer is the one with the vote. As a general rule, however, we attain a remarkable degree of consensus because corporate staff members have a professional respect for their colleagues, enjoy each other's successes, and when you get right down to it, genuinely like each other. There is an astounding amount of regular informal information sharing among members of the corporate Staff. Office-hopping is a widespread corporate habit—a virtue not a vice in our opinion. Seldom, if ever, and then only through exceptional oversight, does a corporate officer get blindsided. That kind of attitude tends to catch-on among the rest of the management team.

Individual corporate staff members make it a regular practice to encourage their department heads to touch base with other department heads on all projects, changes, or activities that affect others. They regularly give them positive or, if necessary, corrective feedback on involving affected managers in the planning and implementation of cross-departmental efforts. During each department head's annual measurable performance review, corporate staff officers discuss their previous year's record of coordination and collaboration and negotiate expectations for cooperation during the next evaluative period. For example, several years ago during my own performance evaluation, Don Creamer expressed his dissatisfaction with the leadership I was providing in coordinating with our nursing department. Beginning soon after and up until today, leaders from nursing and human resources have a working lunch every week to coordinate our activities. That practice has occasioned a phenomenal improvement in our relationship and collaboration. Being a team player does not have pejorative connotations at our place. Being a hot dog does.

Finally, we actively foster CQI work across departmental lines. We especially like to see joint CQI projects among clinical and support departments. In addition to promoting inter-departmental quality initiatives in our criteria for the Chairman's Quality Award Program, vice-presidents are expected to promote such joint initiatives at their divisional meetings, and all managers on all levels are evaluated on their ecumenical approach to quality. This year, as part of our chairman's award program, we have received several joint CQI proposals such as: telecommunications and fiscal services; Utilization review, medical records, and risk management; 4 East, 4 West, ICU, and emergency services.

We hope to promote more frequent combined departmental projects in the years to come.

THE CONTINUITY OF CONTINUOUS QUALITY
IMPROVEMENT: The Fixed Unchanging Target

I have this brilliant theory about how to get dependable participant evaluations on training sessions. The method is reliable and inexpensive. I hope you don't think it's too sneaky. Just go into a rest room after a presentation and listen. I did that several months ago after a talk on reengineering given to the management team of one of the largest hospitals in the country. The presenter essentially said, "CQI is dead. Reengineering is in. Fixing existing systems is never the thing to do. Replacing all systems is the way to go. Ditch improving! Start removing!" One participant summarized the overwhelming reaction of my scientifically selected probability sample when he said: "How can they expect us to be serious about anything when everything is always changing?"

We've got to put the continuity back into continuous quality improvement. Seldom do we need to start from scratch. Starter dough always looks small, inconsequential, and unimportant. Those of us who bake bread know better. Starter dough takes a long time to become activated. But when it's ready, it can leaven a mass of dough much larger than itself. Even the most apparently lifeless institutions possess their starters. They often do not need ever-changing additions of new yeasts. Sometimes, all they need is new bakers who know as much. For example, CQI is essentially the application of the scientific method to the service-improvement process. Physicians are formally trained in and apply the scientific method in their daily practice. The starter is already there. Physicians have got to feel that we CQI "Johnny-Come-Latelys" acknowledge the power of their methods ourselves, the underlying rationale of the quality-improvement task, and are willing to embark on collaborative efforts using a terminology physicians already understand, rather than the imposed jargon, and want to work with them to make things better for our patients.

Every hospital has people who truly care long before formal customer services programs are begun. Every hospital has people trying to make things work more smoothly before the first class is offered on CQI statistical tools. Every hospital has physicians, nurses, and clinicians who have spent their lives trying to make the way they perform a certain procedure, conduct a certain surgery, or supervise a certain regiment a best practice before the first benchmarking CQI group sets out on its quest for the patient management guideline. Continuity in CQI means starting with the semantically different, formally unorganized, and likely uncoordinated but substantially compatible efforts already in place.

Wherever possible, build on what's already there. Stick with the proven mainstays: quality will always be the competitive edge. Managers will always be held accountable for quality results. Employees will always be expected to deliver go-beyond quality along three quality dimensions: C.A.R.E.ing personal service, smooth-running service processes, and positive healthcare results. Along with faith, hope, and charity, these are three examples of the quality things that last. Do variations on the basic popular breads. Introduce new varieties in ways that do not eliminate or reduce the quality of the old favorite standards. Build on what is there. Trim off from what is there—add on to what is there.

At The Williamsport Hospital & Medical Center, we have tried to sustain continuity in our CQI efforts by translating these metaphors into standard operating procedures—by identifying and sticking to the things that last.

6

Making Quality a Habit Through Recognition and Rewards

"Treat people as if they were what they ought to be; and you'll help them become what they are capable of being."

—Goethe

One day, the famous nineteenth century Italian artist Gabrielle Rossetti was approached by an old painter requesting the master's opinion of his work. He let the old man down easily and gently and spent several hours coaching him before their meeting ended. Just before he left, the old man rummaged through his portfolio and extracted a sheave of time-worn sketches. Gabrielle was dumb-struck by their evocative originality. "Who did these?" he demanded. "A Friend? A relative? A student? They're the kind of work from which artistic movements begin." "No," replied the old man, "They are mine. I did them all before I turned twenty. I only wish someone would have noticed then."

Our director of safety and security, Charlie Wolverton, is a master of bringing the best out in people by attending to their growth and applauding their progress. Over the past 10 years, Charlie has put the polish on a half dozen diamonds in the rough who are now highly trained, proud security officers in a safety and security department we'd compare to any other anywhere. He's demanding but fair and takes corrective action whenever necessary. But beyond that, he makes sure solid performance never goes unnoticed. People tend to repeat the things they do that are followed by pleasant consequences. Translating that insight into the way things are done in a business is in our opinion a principal responsibility of management.

MAGIC MOMENT PROGRAM:
Transforming Moments of Truth Into Go-Beyond Encounters

On a harsh winter day several weeks ago, one of our hospital's home health employees, Chris Downey, made a delivery to an elderly woman living alone in a trailer home at a rather remote part of our service area. She had a bad leak in her kitchen ceiling. It wasn't likely, Chris thought, that she could afford to have the snow removed. So, after work that day, Chris drove out to the trailer and cleared the entire roof himself. *That's* a magic moment—an extraordinary one to be sure—one of the close to 10,000 magic moments we've recognized since we began our program seven years ago. To paraphrase the Dean Witter commercial, at The Williamsport Hospital & Medical Center, we measure success one magic moment at a time. Here are but a few examples:

- A patient without a ride to a town called Renovo 60 miles away—an employee drives him there on his own time.
- An elderly terminally ill patient is transferred to a hospice— another employee visits her every day for more than a month until she passes away.
- A poor young mother needs to visit her seriously ill father but cannot leave her sick three year old at home—yet another employee volunteers to babysit.

Here's the way the program works. The idea was simple: anyone could nominate employees, volunteers, or members of our medical staff for a magic moment. (Resource 6-1 shows our magic moments nomination form.) We reward magic moment makers with a lunch on the house and a magic moment button. Three-time winners receive a Celebrate Those Magic Moments T-shirt. Magic moment makers receive other rewards for 10 and 20 magic moments. Employees with 25 magic moments get a day off with pay. In seven years, we have honored our employees for more than 10,000 magic moments.

Resource 6-1. Magic Moments Nomination Form

I would like to bring to your attention a Magic Moment that tran-

spired on _____ at The Williamsport Hospital & Med-
                    (Date)

ical Center. _____ from the
                (Name of employee, volunteer or physician)

_____ Department acted in an exemplary, caring manner and should be recognized.

I am nominating this person because he/she contributed to The Williamsport Hospital & Medical Center's Magic Moments Program in the following way:

(Please be specific. Some examples of Magic Moments are "Helped a coworker change a flat tire," "Escorted a visitor directly to an area rather than giving the visitor directions," "Used off-duty time to comfort and reassure a patient."

_____

_____

_____

_____

_____

_____

_____

This person deserves to have their Magic Moment celebrated.

Name: _____

Signature: _____

Department: _____

Date: _____

Please place completed Magic Moments Nomination Forms in designated Nomination Form boxes or return to the Human Resources Department.

Our magic moment program serves two important purposes. First, magic moment awards provide us with a simple but effective means of fostering and recognizing the daily practice of go-beyond quality among our employees, our medical staff, and our volunteers. Service ideals like go-beyond quality tend to become hollow, rhetorical, and abstract slogans unless organizations find ways of institutionally integrating them into the fabric of the ordinary workday. The magic moment program helps us bridge the gap between our organization's belief system and our employees' service style.

In addition, the magic moment program performs another valuable function. Many of us have not yet been able to make C.A.R.E. a habit, a patterned part of our working lives the way our C.A.R.E. employees of the month have. But all of us strive to emulate the behavior of these C.A.R.E. exemplars and do indeed make some moments of truth magical. These individual encounters need to be applauded and celebrated to encourage all of us to broaden the scope of our work lives that is permeated by the ideal of go-beyond service. William Wordsworth once said: "The best portion of a good man's life—his little nameless unremembered acts of kindness and of love." Through our magic moment program, we name and we remember these acts. Over the years, we have found that doing so is a useful way of succeeding at what Wordsworth has called "the art of getting someone to do something that you want done because he wants to do it."

C.A.R.E. EMPLOYEES OF THE YEAR AND MONTH:
Honoring Those Whom We All Wish to Become

I just can't wait until tomorrow night. It's the night of our ninth annual C.A.R.E. Employee and Physician of the Year Banquet. It is the night on which The Williamsport Hospital & Medical Center celebrates what it wishes to become—a hospital in which everyone is worthy to be a C.A.R.E. employee of the month. (Resource 6-A and 6-B show our C.A.R.E. employee and physician of the month nomination forms.) And do we ever do it up right! The gala event is our equivalent of the Academy Awards.

So far, 216 employees and 46 physicians have joined our C.A.R.E. Hall of Fame. Most still work with us. In fact, one out of every nine of our current employees are C.A.R.E. employees of the month and one out of every 10 of our medical staff are C.A.R.E. physicians of the month. Surprisingly but quite honestly, the caliber of the C.A.R.E. selections is as high as it was nine years ago.

They say that in baseball, you have to do it at least three years in a row before you are what they say you are. There's nothing magical about three years, but the same sort of consistency required of a great hitter over time applies to anyone aspiring to be a member of the Hospital's C.A.R.E. Hall of Fame. We recognize magic moment makers for individual acts of go-beyond quality. We recognize C.A.R.E. employees and physicians of the month for being courteous, attentive, responsive, and empathic steadfastly, as a matter of habit, and over the long-haul. Williamsport is the home of Little League Baseball. Our C.A.R.E. employees and physicians make us the home of Major League Healthcare!

One of the most flattering compliments you can receive from an Italian is to have him say of you that you are *Buono (a) come il pane—* that is, that you are as good as bread. That's about what we think of our C.A.R.E. winners. Each of our C.A.R.E. employees are *Buono (a) come il pane.* Italians also often use the word *companatico* when they refer to any other food that goes well with bread. When you think about it, just about every food goes well with bread and for many, a meal, any meal, is not a meal without bread. Similarly, the way we see things, a service is not a service if it is not suffused with the *c*ourtesy, *a*ttentiveness, *r*esponsiveness and *e*mpathy, the trademark of all of our C.A.R.E. employees and physicians.

THE CHAIRMAN'S QUALITY AWARD:
Even Sinatra Would Be Proud

Players score touchdowns; football teams win championships. Voters cast ballots; constituencies elect candidates. Composers write music; orchestras play symphonies. Soldiers earn medals; nations win wars. Workers put bread on the table; families define societies. Individuals make quality possible; groups of people working together make quality actual.

Our magic moment makers and C.A.R.E. employees and physicians are the ones whose beliefs and work ethic create the culture within which the ideal of go-beyond quality takes root and grows. We constantly honor, thank, and recognize them to help sustain this fertile culture. We direct our magic moment and C.A.R.E. awards toward individuals. But as Casey Stengel has said: "Getting good players is easy. Getting them to play together—that's the hard part." Our Chairman's Quality Award program is one way we try to get all of our staff to do just that—to work together in the pursuit of service excellence. (Resource 6-C presents an overview of the program.)

Here's the way it's working now. Every year, for the last three years, every department in the hospital has been required to design and implement a CQI project in either a key moment of truth in personal service (C.A.R.E.), a quality critical service process (TQM), or a high-volume, high-cost, or problem-prone diagnosis or procedure (MEDIM-PROVE). Corporate staff from the hospital's quality council score and rank submissions according to preset and announced criteria. Resource 6-D provides the details of the 1993 Chairman's Quality Award projects.

The chairman's award program is now in its fifth year. In the first year, we asked departments to develop a service plan including an identification of its principal customers, their customers key moments of truth, their customers requirements during these moments of truth and the methodically planned response we guarantee for each of these customer designated high-priority needs. In the second year, we asked every department to update their service plans and to develop and conduct orientation and training programs to make sure that the plans were translated into action throughout the hospital. We continue to update these service plans every year.

This year we will recognize the best CQI submissions in several stages. First, we will select and reward all of the employees in the top five submissions for each of the three dimensions of quality. A week later, we will announce and give tribute to the top three departments in each of the dimensions of quality. A week after that—the top department in each dimension of quality. And finally, in conjunction with our first annual quality fair, we will select the number-one CQI project of the year.

We at The Williamsport Hospital & Medical Center are proud of our CQI teams' successful quality projects and we want to tell everybody about our employees and what they do to improve our customers' service experiences. So this year we are holding our first annual quality fair. At the fair, 15 CQI teams—the top five finalists in each of the three dimensions of quality (C.A.R.E., TQM, and MEDIMPROVE)— will display storyboards on their award-winning CQI submissions. Our eight cycle of service teams will also display their most influential project. At the fair, we will announce the number-one CQI gold medal award from among the top winners in the C.A.R.E., the TQM, and the MEDIMPROVE categories. We will also make some special CQI recognition awards to selected leaders playing key roles in our overall CQI effort.

We have invited participants in business and industry throughout the community. Our special guests will be representatives from our county's quality-improvement network, which now includes close to 100 businesses. Their effort is aimed at making Lycoming County "Quality County USA." Our hospital is a proud leading member of this communitywide quality-promoting resource and information sharing.

We will also be inviting our partners in quality: the hospital's vendors cooperative venture. Our CEO, Don Creamer, will do the honors at this event. The chairman of our board and a leading business quality advocate and president of a local oil company, Dick DeWald, will present the awards. It's going to be a glorious day. I can't wait.

THE THANK-YOU PLACE: Reviving the *Merenda*

A friend once asked and answered his own rhetorical question: "How am I doing? I don't know. My boss hasn't chewed me out lately."

After close to 10 years of managerial modeling, management training, cajoling, persuading, preaching, and pleading, about 16 percent of our employees—250 in all—still go home every day feeling that what they do is not appreciated. We've got to keep plugging away. We've got to come up with some new ideas. We've got to do better. And we've got to keep up the things we're already doing that have reduced the number of the taken for granted from 500 a decade ago.

One of my favorite ways of making people feel appreciated is what Italians call *merende*. If you asked anyone around here what merende are, I doubt that anyone would know. Before I tell you more about them, I've got to tell you something about my deepest personal beliefs.

To my way of thinking, the most penetrating commentary on human life was made by Virginia Woolf in *A Room of One's Own:*

> "One cannot think well, love well, sleep well
> . . . if one has not dined well."

When I go to a hospital as a patient, my two top demands in order of priority are: fantastic, memorable meals and coming out alive. Merende originated in Italy's rural past. Farmers worked long, tiring days in the field for up to 16 hours too far away from home to return for meals. *Merende* were the varied, irresistibly delicious between-meal meals. In the old days, a *merenda* was usually thickly sliced country bread and whatever else was around and in season: home-cured olives, cheese, walnuts, tuna, anchovies sprinkled with garlic, pepper and a little olive oil, salami, prosciutto—you name it. These simple *merende* eventually became more elaborate and gave birth to the bruschetta, crostini, foccaccia, pizza, and other treats we all enjoy in Italian restaurants.

A *merenda* is work food—any kind of food given to people who work hard and do a good job. In our country, the equivalent can be anything from pizza, doughnuts, a tray of cookies or sandwich meats, a free meal, ice-cream sundae, freshly baked breads—the limits are set only by one's imagination. At The Williamsport Hospital & Medical Center, we use *merende* often as an expression of our appreciation: lunch and banquets for C.A.R.E. employees and physicians, special lunches for CQI team members, pizza parties for magic moment makers, cookie trays for employees celebrating their annual professional weeks, homemade breads and cakes for units or departments working extra-long hours, midnight pizza C.A.R.E. rounds at least once a month for our night-shift employees. *Merende* have three characteristics necessary in any sustainable program for expressing appreciation: they are genuinely appreciated, they are limitlessly varied, and they are affordable.

Years ago, when I worked in another institution, a friend confided: "When my mother died, my world came to an abrupt stop. But at work, things went on as if nothing had happened." People tend not to forget you when you remember to share the times when they grieve and the times when they have something to celebrate. So the corporate staff always sends flowers or food on the occasion of the death of a close relative of employees and makes a point of personally congratulating in writing employees who successfully progress professionally or attain publicly known laudable personal goals.

Within the last month, for example, Eileen Chiama and Nancy Geedey from our occupational health program were accepted as speakers at a national conference in San Diego; three of our rehab LPNs, Joanne Dietrich, Ann Minarsky, and Linda Black, graduated as Physical Therapy Assistants, and Donnie Evans from our dietary department graduated from the STEP Inc. Adult Work Experience Program. We celebrated each happy event with congratulatory letters, a little party, and public notice in the *Centerpiece*. Here's what we had to say about Donnie in our weekly newsletter:

Applause
Congratulations!

Congratulations to **Donnie Evans**. He recently graduated from the Step Inc. Adult Work Experience Program. From a class of 48 participants, Donnie was asked to address the graduates and guests at the ceremonies held on Monday evening at Divine Providence Hospital auditorium. He also was recipient of the Reading Award and the Positive Personality Award.

Donnie Evans is a relatively new Williamsporter and has been working as a cook in our dietary department since November 1993, in conjunction with Step Inc. He is now a hospital employee.

As Bob Nelson explains in *1001 Ways to Reward Employees* (Workman, 1994): "Gratitude is an attitude." We intend all of these gestures and expressions of gratitude to make all of our employees feel that they do indeed work in the thank you place.

LIKE POLITICS, ALL MOTIVATION IS LOCAL:
The Role of the Supervisor

Even in short crash courses on motivation, presenters usually explain and apply the motivational theories of Abraham Maslow and Frederick Herzberg. My observation is that supervisors tend to like Maslow. (See chapter 5 for more in-depth discussion of Maslow and Herzberg.) He's easy to understand and remember and the implications of his theory for supervisory practice are clear and straightforward.

According to Maslow, we all have five levels of human needs. If a motive is a drive toward a goal to satisfy a need, Maslow would say that we are most strongly driven to those goals that satisfy our lowest unfulfilled needs. Maslow calls our lowest level needs basic needs, physiological needs we share with the rest of the animal world—survival needs for water, food, shelter, and air. A hungry penniless illegal immigrant may steal a loaf of bread even if he jeopardizes such higher-level needs as:

- His need for everything that provides basic needs on a predictable basis (security needs like a job and money and benefits a job brings).
- His need to be accepted (belonging needs).
- His need to feel recognized and appreciated (ego-status needs).
- His need to be his very best self (self-actualization needs).

Maslow's advice to supervisors: discover the current unmet needs of individual employees and motivate them by appealing to these unmet needs. Maslow's insight has been translated into the so-called platinum rule: treat others the way *they* (not necessarily *you*) want to be treated. This twist on the golden rule forces supervisors to break their one-size-fits-all motivational paradigm, to intensify their communication with employees to discern individual needs, and to "particularize" their motivational strategies.

Several years ago, a supervisor recommended disciplining a young employee by suspending him for a day without pay. The youngster lived with parents who indulged his every wish. The employee let it be known he would appreciate an extra day off. The suspension was promised on the belief that he needed the money. He didn't. The employee's unmet need was additional leisure time, not additional pay. After some discussion with the supervisor, we decided to make the employee work an extra day on a weekend. In reverse, Maslow had struck with a vengeance!

Maslow goes down easily with supervisors because he spreads the job of motivating throughout all levels of management. Herzberg is a different story. When he gets finished explaining his two-factor theory the motivational buck stops on top of the front-line supervisor's desk.

In my adapted version of Herzberg's theory, Maslow's two lowest need levels are called novocaine factors. Herzberg calls them hygiene factors. In business organizations, these need levels include wages and benefits. The ability to affect these needs resides in top management. By fulfilling these lower level needs, companies temporarily reduce dissatisfaction. They take away the pain. Once removed, the pain returns—because improvements in wages and benefits soon become entitlements. They do not motivate over the long term. For the most part, compensation packages in hospitals are pretty competitive.

In my version of the Herzberg model, the top three levels of need (belonging, ego-status, and self-actualization) are called turn-ons. Herzberg calls them motivators. We agree with Herzberg that there are human values beyond profit to which people are willing to dedicate their efforts. I remember asking an especially caring go-beyond nurse a year or so ago what made her extend herself so far beyond what was necessary. She responded: "In their own quiet way, my patients always let me know that what I do for them makes a big difference in their lives, that what I do is important. I like to feel needed." In most business settings, the ability to appeal to employees through the fulfillment of these higher-level needs resides not in top management, but to some degree in middle management, and to a very substantial degree in front-line supervisors and sometimes, as in this example, in our patients. As Tim Allen would say, "That's where the pinion meets the fly wheel," or in non-*Home Improvement* jargon, "where the rubber meets the road." Over time, it's the way the quality mission, value, and quality goals of an organization transform service encounters into episodes of legendary service.

Tip O'Neill used to say: "All politics is local." Similarly we think all motivation is local. Supervisors who frequently perceive themselves as impotent, actually have within their command and control the most potent means to inspire employees to practice go-beyond quality. Successful supervisors are those who perform the one-minute manager's ABCs of management (*a*ctivating through goal setting, coaching and facilitating *b*ehavior and managing the *c*onsequences of performance) in ways that get people to feel they belong and are really somebody and feel free to be all that they can be. In *1001 Ways to Reward Employees,*

Bob Nelson make a good case for this point: "Psychological paychecks have an intrinsic value that hard currency can never touch." You wouldn't think that having a particular boss would make much difference to main switchboard operators at the hospital. But it does. Just last week, employees were anticipating new organizational reporting relationships, I was deluged with this request: "Whatever happens, please don't take Charlie away from us." Supervisors like Charlie who get employees to achieve institutional quality ideas by satisfying high-level employee needs establish the vital link between what an organization wants and what workers want. They are aligning the personal and professional aspirations of employees and organization's goals.

The winningest coach in the history of college football, Bear Bryant, used to ask every single player on his team to write out his personal goals. He made a point of developing the team's season strategy only after he had read them all. In this way, Bryant effectively told his players that he cared about them and their desires and that on his team, players could pursue their own goals and that their goals were part of the team's plan. His record is ample proof of how well this technique worked. Effective supervisors know it works off the playing field as well. I'd like to say that Coach Bryant's approach to goal setting prevails at The Williamsport Hospital & Medical Center, but it doesn't—not yet at least. I plan to implement the coach's idea this year with our human resources staff. After a year's experience, I intend to integrate Coach Bryant's approach into our management training.

APPRECIATION REVIEWS: A Renewal of Vows

Several years ago, I attended the twenty-fifth wedding anniversary of some friends of mine. Theirs had been a happy marriage as marriages go, but not without some tough times. At a short church service, they renewed their marriage vows. The day was a celebration of their good times together; they had long since worked through the not-so-good times. The day was a promise of hope for their future years together; the past was irretrievably gone and not within their power to refashion.

We think annual performance evaluations motivate employees to do quality work if evaluations share these features of a renewal of marriage vows. First, they ought to be a celebration of past successes. They ought to be appreciation reviews. They ought to focus more on planning the next evaluation period than in rehashing the past, especially past failures.

The following sections discuss our deeply held beliefs that underscore this view of performance evaluations:

The most important aspect of performance evaluation is regular, timely feedback on the results of an employee's work.

The supervisor's job is to serve as an institutional thermostat. When employees are doing well, their performance ought to be maintained through positive reinforcement. When employees fail to meet quality standards, supervisors need to intervene correctively and constructively to return performance back to a pre-set standard.

We have just completed an audit of performance evaluations for the last quarter of the year. Twenty-eight employees did not meet all of the key expectations of their job. They are automatically on a 90-day probation period. Their situation: get your performance up to our standards with our help or face progressive punitive discipline like suspension and termination.

Feedback ought to be positive when possible and corrective only when necessary.

In many places, the vast majority of employees do things well the vast majority of the time. Too often, in those same places, the most prevalent form of managerial feedback is often critical, not constructively critical. As Ken Blanchard says: "Positive feedback is the breakfast of champions."

We evaluate our evaluations. This year, for example, 92 percent of our managers and supervisors who received a favorable evaluation, felt good about the evaluation they received. That's up from 64 percent eight years ago—but we still have a way to go.

The one-minute praising and the one-minute reprimand ought to be a memorized tool in the repertoire of every supervisor.

They are the most rudimentary form through which the consequences of behavior are managed. One of the standard questions on the final exam of our basic managerial leadership course—yes, we have a final combination written and verbal exam and yes sometimes people fail—is to give the steps and a real life example of a one-minute praising and a one-minute reprimand.

Here are examples two managers gave in a recent written exam after completing our Management Leadership Course:

One-Minute Praising

1. Mary, I'd like to talk to you about the way you handled that angry group of visitors yesterday afternoon.
2. You couldn't have done a better job.
3. When they loudly complained about the end of visiting hours, you led them to our conference room out of earshot, let them vent, got them calmed down and actually got them to listen to your explanation about time limits on visiting.
4. I was beaming with pride about your finesse. The other staff were relieved about the conclusion of an awkward confrontation. Patients and family members saying goodbye breathed a sigh of comfort. Dr. Eshelman complemented me about your performance.
5. I'll tell you Mary, it's great to know I have someone like you on board to help with the difficult situations we sometimes encounter. Thanks. Great job!

One-Minute Reprimand

1. Bill, I'd to talk to you about the patient pick-up of Mr. Johns this morning. I've spoken to you and everyone involved.
2. I've got serious problems with what you did.
3. You were supposed to bring Mr. Johns up for surgery. You went to the wrong room, walked in and announced "Johns?" The patient there was John Smith. He was on medication and answered "Yes." Against his and his family's protests, you insisted he was scheduled for surgery. He was not. You didn't check—not even his name band!
4. Mr. Smith and his family were appalled. They're spreading the word to others about your flagrant abandonment of required

procedures, tact, and courtesy. I'm mortified. Your colleagues are embarrassed. The incident is a horrible contradiction of our standards of care—no mind that backup procedures would have discovered your error and no physical harm would have been done.

5. After discussing this with Human Resources, I've decided to suspend you for three days without pay. If any similar incident occurs, you could be subject to termination. Bill, this just isn't like you. I'm sure that in the future, you will continue to practice the dependability and good judgment I've always known you model.

Annual performance reviews ought to be an exchange of information, not a report card.

Though final evaluative decisions are the supervisor's prerogative, they should be based on the most complete available information, including the perspective of the employee being evaluated. For this reason, whether the evaluation is initiated by the person evaluated as a self-evaluation or by the supervisor—the other is required to react to the original evaluation and personally discuss both perspectives in developing the final result.

Annual performance reviews ought to be summaries, not surprises.

Because effective supervisors give regular feedback, it is superfluous to go over old ground except in a summary fashion, to celebrate the mountain of good work and to move on to plan the future having learned the little molehill of work that needs to be improved. We've gotten really good at this. It's taken time, but this year only 4 percent of our managers and supervisors said they were surprised by the feedback they received in their performance evaluations.

Every employee has the right to regular feedback.

All employees can expect a competently conducted, thorough, fair, and constructive annual performance evaluation.

The purpose of performance evaluations is to enhance future performance.

A substantial part of the evaluation interview should be spent on planning. We use the following formula as a flexible guideline. Evaluations are a time to RAP:

- *R* = *R*eview—spend up to 20 percent of the interview time on reviewing past performance.
- *A* = *A*ssess—spend about the same amount of time assessing progress and the current state of performance. Reward progress, not just perfection.
- *P* = *P*lan—spend 50 percent to 60 percent of the time on planning the future.

We've been spending time in training recently teaching managers to extract the future implications of their reviews of past performance. It's a difficult skill to learn and a difficult skill to teach.

Employees who receive an overall positive rating ought to feel they received a positive evaluation when it is all over.

In the evaluations we do of our personnel evaluations, that—surprisingly—does not always happen.

Bad things can happen after poorly done reviews, even if they are done with the best of intentions. Sometime back, one of our managers tried to improve the behavior of a problem employee by giving the employee an excellent performance review and rating. The employee was a technically good performer but was a divisive and manipulative group member. When the destructive impact of the employee's behavior could no longer be ignored, the necessary intervention became more complicated than would otherwise have been the case. Not too long ago, another manager who prides himself on being a tough scorer, did a hatchet job on an excellent employee to bring out her full potential. When this employee applied for a position in another department, her evaluation ruined her chances and the job went to a much less qualified candidate.

CORRECTIVE INTERVENTION:
Going Against the Manager's Personal Grain

As *The One Minute Manager* (Berkley Books, 1984) reminds us, leave-alone-zap has become the most prevalent style of management in the United States. Anyone in human resources can tell you what leave-alone-zap is. An outraged manager storms into human resources bellowing for all to hear that Perpetua Ineptitude ought to be terminated today—right now. Truth is, the manager is often right. Then we look at Ms. Ineptitude's previous evaluations. "Exceeded expectations," they usually say. "Okay, have you given her feedback? Have you documented her performance deficiencies? Have you worked with her to bring her up to snuff? Have you progressively disciplined her?" No, all the supervisor has done is left her alone. The saga of Perpetua Ineptitude would be really funny if it were not so common place.

Unfortunately, the leave-alone part of the practice usually goes on for a long, long time. Tolerating substandard performance brings to the highest level of visibility the truth that the organization rewards behavior about which it should be mortified. Employees hear the business preach quality and watch it practice a tolerance for mediocrity and even inferiority.

We spend a lot of time telling our supervisors that they are the only ones who can make our corporate value—C.A.R.E. for our employees and for our customers—come alive. We want our supervisors to be flexible on most things but very hard on our values. This mandate requires them to intervene to improve the performance of employees falling short of the C.A.R.E. standard. A receptionist projects an attitude of indifference; a manager frequently upbraids his employees in the presence of others; a caregiver's attempt at humor comes across as caustic and uncaring to patients; an exempt manager punches a clock when her continued presence is necessary to take care of our patients' needs. These kinds of behaviors contradict our value of go-beyond C.A.R.E. These employees have a right to feedback that will help them improve, a right to help to improve, a right to time to improve. They do not have a right to fail to improve. After every reasonable effort fails to change the performance, we expect supervisors to work fairly to change the person. Our only choices are to get people up to our quality standards, and that failing, to get quality people to take their place. As we have said before, you can't have total quality without total quality managers.

"SO YOU DON'T LIKE IT HERE?":
Separating the Culturally Antagonistic

We service providers are getting more than our share of people coming to work for us who are simply not nice to each other and to our customers and not very motivated to do their best by their co-workers and our customers. At best, they are indifferent. We call these employees the culturally antagonistic. They kill a place's chances of growing quality by contaminating the environment in which quality thrives. We try hard to avoid hiring them. We try hard to change them if we mistakenly bring them on board. We aggressively but fairly terminate their employment if we fail to bring them around. Over the years, our managers have gotten progressively better at being willing to swiftly deal with our cultural misfits—the antitheses of go-beyond quality.

We train all of our managers on how to deal with the employee and the problem manager. We define problem employees as those whose patterned performance in either the task dimension or the relational dimension of their job seriously and adversely affects either our customers' satisfaction or our employees' morale.

In the past year, we have intervened to correct or eliminate task deficiencies like chronic absenteeism and tardiness, an exceptional instance of medication errors, the recalcitrant violation of our appearance code, a lackadaisical response pattern to answering patient bills, theft, and falsification of time records. We have also stepped in to hand relational shortcomings in performance like failure to use the magic phrases ("please," "thank you," "you're welcome," "I'm sorry," people's names), improper or discourteous telephone answering, failure to acknowledge, smile at, and greet people, and violation of any of the other C.A.R.E. behaviors. We teach supervisors how to apply the hot stove theory so that employees who touch our value stove receive warnings when they're close and get burned as soon as they touch it. We expect managers to deliver a one-minute reprimand the very first time employees deviate from the hospital's task and relational expectations—before an unacceptable pattern of undesirable behavior is established. We teach the educational meaning of discipline: how to work with problem employees to improve their performance. We expect managers to do more than point out what is wrong with an employee's performance. We expect them to teach, show, and model what is right and to give employees feedback as well as the time and the help necessary to improve. Finally, we teach supervisors the punitive meaning of discipline: how to work with our employee relations director to apply progressive forms of punishment—including suspension and termination—if the requirements of customer enthusiasm and employee morale call for it. When preventative and corrective discipline fail, we do not hesitate to apply punitive discipline, including termination. When we can't change the behavior, we change the person—regrettably more than 250 in the last 10 years. Hospitals that C.A.R.E. about their patients and their employees fire employees who don't.

Our employees are doubting Thomas' and Thomasina's. St. Thomas said: "Unless I see . . ., I will not believe." Our employees, too, say: "Show me." Show me that you recognize go-beyond quality in magic moments. Show me that you put quality C.A.R.E. exemplars on a pedestal. Show me that you reward group quality work. Show me that you're proud of our quality successes and are willing to show them off. Show me that you appreciate us when we treat our fellow employees and patients well. Show me that my work life will be fulfilling because you'll make sure I have a good supervisor. Show me that you won't put up with sloppy work. Show me you won't tolerate employees who are a mockery to everything we stand for. In the words of the memorable tune from *My Fair Lady:* "Don't talk of love, show me." When all of these things are transparently visible, I'll show you a quality place.

7

Human Resources: The Key to Quality Service

> "Organizations exist to serve the needs of the
> people who are serving the customer."

—Karl Albrecht and Ron Zemke, *Service America*

After years of success at providing quality products and service, pleasing his customers, maintaining a happy and productive workforce and running a financially successful company, the president of a family-owned business turned over the reins to his eldest son. The new president immediately launched a flurry of radical changes including reorganization and layoffs. Morale dipped. Product and service quality fell. The company started showing red on its bottom line for the first time in its long history. The son asked his father for some advice. One afternoon soon after, the father took his son out in a rowboat on a quiet lake. Once they got to the middle, the father handed over the oars to his son and instructed him to row with only one oar. They began to go around in circles. Then the father told his son to row only with the other oar. Naturally the same thing happened again.

Finally, the father said this: "Son, running a business is like rowing a boat. You've got to use both oars. The one oar is your employees. The other oar is your customers. The secret to success is simple: **you take care of your employees and they will take care of your customers.**"

If you were to ask the management staff at any hospital throughout the country whether they firmly believed in the moral of this story, 100 percent of them would probably answer yes. If you were to ask the employees of all of the hospitals in the country whether their management teams acted as though they believed in the moral of this story, how many hospitals do you think would get a resounding positive response? Whatever the number, I'd be inclined to want to go to the ones with a positive employee ratings for my healthcare needs. I'd lay down money that they are as good with their patients as they are with their employees.

In a hospital, the calling of a caregiver is to keep or make customers well and happy. The calling of the management team is to enable and motivate caregivers to *want* to keep or make customers happy—to increase the institution's ability to achieve its quality mission by integrating individual desires for growth and development with organizational goals. The customer is the final arbiter of service quality. Employees are the final arbiter of managerial quality. To paraphrase Karl Albrecht: The single most important measure of management quality is the quality of management as perceived by employees compared to their own expectations and hopes.

In 1985, when The Williamsport Hospital & Medical Center asked its employees whether they agreed with this statement: "The Williamsport Hospital & Medical Center really values its employees," 43 percent said no. In 1993-94, when we asked our employees the same question, eight percent of them said no. 92 percent said yes. In a year when our employee dental and vision plans were eliminated, when 156 employees had their hours reduced from 40 hours a week to 37.5 hours a week, when our cafeteria subsidy was drastically reduced, and when a consolidation with a former competitor augured the imminent elimination of some jobs, 92 percent of our employees said they thought we valued them. Here's why we think it happened.

PEOPLE PRODUCE QUALITY SYSTEMS AND OUTCOMES:
Employee Morale as the Flip Side of Customer Enthusiasm

My favorite attraction at Disney World's Epcot Center is Cranium Command. Cranium Command is a delightful multimedia show that explains the relationship between the body and the mind in a 12-year-old boy. You see, I'm a sucker for the underdog—any underdog, and in this show, the underdog wins out. In Cranium Command, one subplot is: Who really makes this wondrous specimen function so wonderfully?

The cardiovascular system pontificates: "I make it all happen. Clog me with fa(s)t food and see how you make out!" The neurological system throws down the gauntlet: "Yeh? Try to do it without my infrastructure and communicating systems!" The respiratory system chimes in: "Hey guys, how would you like the oxygen supply cut off—right now?"

After the prestigious anatomical systems have their say, a little six-centimeter-wide organ located at the stem of the brain modestly describes its contribution to the well-being of the 12 year old. It is the hypothalamus. And here is what the hypothalamus does: controls the maintenance of water, balance, sugar and fat metabolism, the regulation of body temperature, the secretion of endocrine glands, the integration of sympathetic and parasympathetic activities, the source of some crucial hormones, and more. Easily overlooked, the hypothalamus is a big-time player and an unsung hero!

So, too, are employees in high-quality service business. In too many places they've got to surrender the spotlight to systems, processes, CQI process tools, clinical pathways, and now, hot shots on the block like reengineering. The all too obvious fact of life is that all of these attention-getting tools and processes never get to happen without quality people any more than the major anatomical transportation systems get to work without the direction of their anatomical traffic cop, the hypothalamus.

Behind our surgeons, physicians, and other high-profile caregivers are a supporting cast of our big little people. Last quarter, 95 percent of our patients rated our environmental service aides as always courteous; 5 percent as usually courteous—that thanks to a department full of people like Dave Mitchley and Olive Miller. In March, we gave out over 400 snow-related magic moments because of a maintenance department with people like Jack Corson, Paul Stetts, Dave Howe, and Jerry Weaver. Over the last half year, we have virtually eliminated complaints related to busy signals in our billing office because people like Connie McFadden and Avie Thompson in our cashier's office and Ruth Pratt and Gloria McDermott in our telecommunications office made the systems and practice changes necessary to achieve this result.

In an article, Dr. Stephen Covey and Keith Gulledge (*Journal for Quality and Participation,* July/August, 1992) drew the connection I am making between employee morale and service quality. "The number-one restraining force to quality," they conclude, "is trust in senior management by employees." A study done several years ago by the Epic

Healthcare Group defined employee commitment in this way: Employees with high levels of commitment to the company believe that:

- Hospital management is interested in their welfare.
- Hospital management is committed to providing quality patient care.
- The hospital lives up to its own guiding principles.
- Communication about what is going on in the hospital is effective.
- Work is interesting and satisfying.

The study concluded that how people feel about their employer makes a big difference not just in morale or satisfaction but also in financial performance and in customer satisfaction—in the perceived quality of the service.

THE HUMAN RESOURCES GOAL:
Employees United in the Pursuit of CQI

An observer at a medieval construction site approached several masons separately and asked: "What are you doing?" The first mason said: "I'm making a living. It's not the greatest job in the world, but it puts bread on the table." The second mason responded: "I'm trying to advance my career and receive recognition within my profession; so I'm going to make the wall I'm working on better built and more beautiful than the others." The third mason answered by saying: "We're building a magnificent cathedral."

The first mason doesn't see any purpose to his work beyond his own personal survival needs. The second mason's goal is higher up on the Maslow hierarchy, but it's still purely individualistic. His relationship to others on the site is competitive, not collaborative. Neither the first nor the second mason see their work as a service to the structure's intended users—future worshippers. The third mason sees himself as a member of a team doing his very best together with the rest to create a place of worship that will serve worshippers for centuries.

Like other service businesses, hospitals have their share of worker type 1, the money grubber and worker type 2, the self-promoter. These kinds of workers do not consistently provide go-beyond service. They are too self-absorbed and self-serving. In a go-beyond service culture, the values, the management style, the customer-focused expectations, and the rewards and punishments make the money grubber and the self-promoter feel out of place. They either change or one way or the other, they leave. They simply do not belong and they soon realize that fact. Go-beyond service businesses do all they can to hire, develop, reward, and promote workers unified in the pursuit of continuous quality improvement.

Some approaches to managing people promote the development of the money grubbers and the self-promoters. Service businesses that place too much emphasis on money or benefits as the most important forms of carrots and sticks tend to attract and retain employees who are like baseball players who are more interested in their own personal statistics than in the whole team's performance. Businesses that place too much emphasis on supporting the self-promotional aspirations of certain professions to the detriment of customer service and value tend to create type-2 employees.

In hospitals, one such familiar practice is to accept only superfluous, educational degrees required by professional associations instead of demonstrated competence as the preferred entry level for a job (for example, the preference of any nurse with a bachelor's degree in nursing for head nurse positions over tried, proven, super-competent, non-degreed nurses who have done the job superlatively already). Hospitals that impose entry hurdles that are not bona fide requirements attract profession-focused, as opposed to customer-focused, employees and de-motivate CQI unifiers by rewarding the ladder climbers.

In accordance with the behavior-based Model of interviewing, described later in this chapter, we follow a three-step process in identifying the candidate best suited for a given position:

- Develop an up-to-date job description.
- Identify and rank the skills required to do the job.
- Ask open-ended questions about past job-related experience in which candidates have demonstrated their relative ability in the skill areas required by the new job.

In filling several directorships of clinical departments in the last few years, we have chosen candidates with proven managerial skills in unrelated departments over candidates with clinical degrees in the specialty but no history of superior managerial performance. Some hospitals still prefer CEOs with medical degrees. We prefer CEOs with a track record of successful leadership as chief executive officers whether or not they are M.D.s. In a word, our interest is in the degree of our employees' demonstrated competence not the number of sheepskins they can hang up in their offices.

We have come to believe that this I-can-do-it-because-I-already-have-done-it approach keeps the doors of promotional opportunity open to all of the potentially qualified. Our practice certainly does not disqualify the qualified the way degree-fixated approaches do. Our practice is inclusive and it unifies. And as we have said before, Employees unified in the pursuit of service excellence form the bridge between what Karl Albrecht calls "the customer value package" and what we call go-beyond value.

EMPLOYEE MORALE IN 1985: A Failing Score

August 8, 1984, was my first day on the job as the new vice-president for human resources at The Williamsport Hospital & Medical Center. So bright and early that morning, I made my way to the employee cafeteria to launch a new era of employee relations. I got my breakfast, walked over, and sat down at the first table with an open chair. Three employees from our maintenance and engineering department—they are now good friends of mine—were engaged in a lively discussion over breakfast. When I sat down, silence. For 20 minutes, despite some ice-breaking efforts on my part, they ignored me! During the next two days, at the same time, I came back again. Same employees, same thing—silence. I was determined to go back as often as it was going to take. Finally, on the fourth day, after pouring a box of cereal into my bowl, one of them passed me the sugar without my even asking! It may have been my imagination, but to this day, I think he smiled. It wasn't a roaring start, but it was a start.

In those days, employee cynicism and distrust ran deep and wide. The next month, when we began our monthly C.A.R.E. Pizza rounds with free pizza, fresh fruit, and sodas for the night shift, the conversation was: "Who's this guy?" "What's he looking for?" "The new corporate people are spying even on the third shift. Watch out?" It took some time before the conversations took on a more friendly tone: "What do ya mean, no pepperoni!"

When we did our first employee climate assessment in late 1984 and early 1985, we weren't exactly expecting canonization by acclamation. But neither were we expecting castigation and condemnation. Some might say the latter is exactly what we got. Let's be kind and just say that the results didn't constitute a strong vote of confidence.

Employees responding to a cluster of eight items affected predominately by mid-level, front-line supervisors, gave our department heads and supervisors a failing grade of 64 percent. Senior management didn't do much better. Employees responding to another cluster of items affected predominately by the corporate staff gave us a failing score of 67 percent. Overall, employee ratings came to a failing score of 69 percent. When asked whether we really valued our employees, we all got a joint failing score of 57 percent. Ever the optimist, I remember thinking: Well, one good thing . . . there's room for improvement! The job was going to be a marathon not a sprint race.

REENGINEERING THE HUMAN RESOURCES SYSTEMS:
Transformation to a Culture That Supports CQI

Culture is a big buzzword these days. It should be. It's not just a passing fad. Culture alone ensures sustained quality. But just what is a culture? The definition given by James Davison Hunter to society at large in *Before the Shooting Begins: Searching for Democracy in America's Culture War* (The Free Press, 1994) serves well as a definition for culture within the organizations: "Culture is first and foremost, a normative order by which we comprehend ourselves, others, and the larger world and through which we order our experience." As author Richard John Neuhaus says: "Culture provides the terms for deciding what is right, what is wrong, what is noble and what is base, what is good and what is evil."

The palpable sign of a quality culture is a workforce united in the pursuit of continuous quality improvement. A quality culture with a big *C* requires a management and employee group characterized by four little *c*s: caring, competence, cooperativeness, and commitment. Such an employee complement is the result of a successful partnership between an institution's management staff and its human resources department. It takes competent, caring, enthusiastic service providers to continuously improve customer-oriented service systems. In a lot of places, the establishment of such a culture is not a matter of improving existing human resources strategies and systems. It is a matter of a radical, fundamental replacement in the jargon of the day, a matter of reengineering.

The following sections describe the seven systems that need to be working well to ensure the creation and maintenance of a culture where quality feels at home.

Systems that ensure the corporate staff and human resources staff model quality service to the hospital's employees.

The human resources department has to set the standard as a service department. The corporate staff has to be the exemplary team builders and team leaders. Human resources and the corporate staff must listen to their customers and respond in a go-beyond way. They say it's got to start at the top. Believe me, on this one, they got it right. Maureen Karstetter sits on the corporate staff as the director of the hospital's foundation. She has every excuse not to be involved in CQI, but Maureen is one of our most faithful participants. Last month, our CFO, Mike Scherneck initiated a write-off of some charges for a patient with a legitimate complaint about the personal service she received. "We didn't give her her money's worth," was the way Mike put it. Our vice-president for medical affairs, Joe English, deals gently but efficiently with problems involving physicians on all dimensions of quality. If you're a physician who was rude to a patient or employee, for example, look forward to seeing Joe.

Systems that ensure management leadership that fosters quality work.

This one is the most important. The degree to which service achieves its full potential is the degree to which managers serve their employees. We like to see our corporate staff and management staff serve food to our volunteers at their annual banquet and serve treats to our employees at the handful of employee thank-you days we have each year. In their leadership training, we teach our managers that the word that comes closest to explaining the words managers and supervisor is *servant*. As we saw in chapter 3, the servant manager keeps all 10 promises in the C.A.R.E. leadership pledge.

Systems that ensure all departments hire first-rate staff.

Resource 7-1 shows our hiring guidelines. We tell all of our new employees that we expect our hospital to be better their first day than it was the day before because they are there. Human resources staff members conduct first-contact screening. We emphasize the primacy of first-hand experience of demonstrated competence over good interviews. We provide intensive orientations that emphasize what we value above all else: our patients and our employees.

Back-up systems through which we can confirm the correctness of our hiring decisions.

The behavior-based model is good but not perfect. Employee certification provides a way to rectify hiring mistakes. We believe in short courtships when our first impression argues against the prospects of a long marriage. When you fail the compulsories in figure skating, you don't get a chance to show off your free-style. When you fail as a probationary employee at The Williamsport Hospital & Medical Center, you never get a chance to enjoy the status of regular employee.

Systems that enable the institution to regularly discern the way employees feel about important aspects of their work life within the hospital.

Our impact statement system, our regular organizational climate assessments (discussed later in this chapter), our open appointment policy (any employee calls any manager at any level and an appointment time is guaranteed) and our open doors—all these practices are intended to say to our employees: What you think matters. Feel free to share it without fear of any adverse consequences.

Resource 7-1. The Williamsport Hospital & Medical Center Hiring and Promotion Guidelines

The culture we wish to establish within The Williamsport Hospital & Medical Center is one that promotes go-beyond patient care and a united workforce that make that level of quality possible. As the alliance value statement says: "What matters most to us are those who receive our care and those who provide our care."

The correct kinds of hiring and promotional policies and practices foster the maintenance of this customer- and employee-focused culture.

CONSEQUENTLY, THE WILLIAMSPORT HOSPITAL & MEDICAL CENTER REQUIRES HIRING THE MOST QUALIFIED AVAILABLE PERSON WHENEVER A POSITION COMES OPEN.

The three basic criteria for hiring and promotion are excellent performance in one's current job, possession of the required skills to do the new job, and length of service. The alliance makes hiring and decisions primarily on the basis of the demonstrated past performance of applicants. When two or more applicants demonstrate comparable performance levels in their current jobs and comparable potential to do the new job, length of service will be considered.

Purpose	To ensure the application of The Williamsport Hospital & Medical Center's principles and policies on hiring and promotion.
Principle 1:	Demonstrated competence is the only bona fide occupational qualification for any and all positions.
Principle 2:	When legally mandated licensure, certification, or registration is required to qualify a candidate for a specific position, this requirement will become an additional bona fide occupational qualification for all candidates.
Principle 3:	We cannot initiate or maintain any policy practice that has the effect of disqualifying the qualified.

Practical Application: Hiring supervisor must write job description and make employment-related decisions using objective skill requirements as the bottom line.

Resource 7-1.   The Williamsport Hospital & Medical Center Hiring and Promotion Guidelines *(continued)*

Further Understanding:

1. The 1978 Uniform Guidelines on Employee Selection Proce-dures, and EEO law, stipulates that the criteria established to select employees must not have an adverse effect on the employment opportunities of any protected class or they are considered to be discriminatory and therefore, illegal. The only exception to the rule is if requirements can be justified by business necessity.

2. Customer, employer or employee preference does not qualify as a business necessity.

3. "Ability to perform" as it relates to educational requirements: A job's educational requirements are not within bonafide occu-pational qualifications exceptions unless it can be shown there is factual basis for believing that all, or substantially all, of the excluded group would be unable to perform the job.

4. The possession of a degree is not presumptive evidence of the superior professional competence of the person with a degree over another without a degree. We are interested in degree of competence not academic degrees except to the extent that they can be successfully argued to enhance competence.

5. The area under Required Education on the job description would state the minimum legal and Alliance identified stan-dards only. Educational preferences are acceptable as long as they are not used to exclude otherwise qualified candidates from consideration and selection. Any approved educational preferences must include the acceptability of demonstrated competence by equivalent experience.

6. Only the Vice President for Human Resources can approve a requirement or preference of an educational degree for any position.

Systems that ensure fairness and consistency in hiring, promotions, rewards, discipline, terminations, and all other human resources transactions.

In 95 percent of cases, we do all of these things in a squeaky clean way. But here, only perfection suffices. Here, it's no defects. So here, we've still got a way to go.

Systems that integrate human resources and the organization's CQI effort.

Human resources functions like recruitment, employment, wages and salary administration, employee relations and training are not meant merely to serve narrow human resources objectives like low vacancy rates, EEOC compliance, the avoidance of compression in compensation, the prevention of union organizing efforts, or the show of organizational erudition. Human resources functions should all be directed at helping our managers to motivate and enable our people to work as individuals and as teams—to create a workforce united in the pursuit of go-beyond quality. Every time the human resources staff is faced with a decision, one question that must always be asked is: How will this affect our employees' ability and desire to do a world-class job together for our customers?

In the rest of this chapter, I will describe the important features and characteristics of each of these systems.

HUMAN RESOURCES DEPARTMENT SERVICES:
Model of Go-Beyond Service

The president of a manufacturing plant was explaining how automation was going to revolutionize his employees' work and their work setting. He described how much of what employees currently did would soon be done by computers and robots. "I realize," he told them, "that many of you are concerned about your jobs. Let me assure you, you will all remain employed. You will have to come in only on Wednesday and because of our increased productivity, we will still pay you for an entire week. Any questions?" he concluded. "Yes," called out one of the employees, "do we have to come in *every* Wednesday?"

Getting away with the barely passable is a way of life with too many employees in our country. One of the blessings of my job is that I am surrounded by people in our human resources department with just the opposite attitude about their work. They expend themselves to the limits of their discretionary efforts. Things like the following happen often:

- Employees have remarked that Jen Mitchell, my secretary, should get an award for the special touch and personal investment she brings to our employee recognition dinners. Jen is one of our C.A.R.E. employees of the month.
- Debbie Loner, our employment manager, frequently baby-sits the children of job candidates from out of town in her own home—sometimes overnight. Debbie also always gives prospective candidates her home telephone number so that if they have any question, they can feel free to call her in confidence in the privacy of their home in the evening. She was a C.A.R.E. employee of the year in 1988.
- In response to a whimsical throwaway about how great a doughnut would taste, our director of employee relations, Dave Heiney, headed out in the midst of a snow storm to bring two dozen doughnuts to the tired staff on a nursing unit. Dave's also always on hand to counsel employees experiencing the traumatic personal and professional problems and tragedies that are a daily part of the life of our 1,500-member hospital family.
- Our receptionist, Bonnie Cole, has the busiest phone in the hospital—bar none. Whether you call her at 8:00 A.M. or 4:30 P.M., you'll still hear the perfect way a phone should be answered. Bonnie was chosen as a C.A.R.E. employee of the year in 1987.
- Through the very special treatment and service provided to them by one of our personnel assistants, Joyce Schramm, our retirees continue to feel like important members of the hospital family.
- Another of our secretaries, Carol Roy, gives one-hour service on information requests from employees seeking mortgages or child subsidies.

- Our policy requires a completed job description before job posting. Sometimes harried managers needing an immediate posting, don't have the time to work one up. Personnel assistant Marilyn Geist, makes the time and does it for them.
- Our compensation manager, Kathy Allen, can often be seen going through a shoe-box of claim forms and bills to help straighten out healthcare insurance claims gone awry.
- We all deliver training programs on whatever shifts to whomever shows up, regardless of the numbers, rather than ask employees to come in when they're off from work.
- Human resources staff members have taken on monthly C.A.R.E. pizza rounds in the wee hours of the morning for the night shift for almost 10 years.

Our Human Resources staff realizes that everyone's most important function is employee relations. Employee titles can detract from their understanding of their key role. In many human resources departments, the position of director of employee relations indicates that employee relations is the domain of the director and not the key element in every human resources staff member's job. At The Williamsport Hospital & Medical Center no one in human resources works under that misconception.

Each member of our human resources department would be the first to admit that we have a long way to go to become a model of go-beyond quality to others in the hospital. Some departments may surpass us in their exercise of legendary service. But whatever shortcomings human resources staff have is a function of our limitations, not of our effort or of our conviction that we, more than anyone, must treat our employees the way we ask them to treat our patients— like gold.

THE RIGHT TO A GOOD MANAGER: A Guaranteed Benefit

Imagine your being hospital vice-president for a day. An employee comes to you and says: "We've got a great department. Our department head is terrific. All of our supervisors are super. The only problem is our customers keep complaining about our service, our employees don't really do a good job, and they sure are unhappy. Morale is terrible!" "Wait a minute," you're saying. "This conversation is whacky. It would never happen." You are right. Good managers are defined by the competent performance of their employees and by the subjective satisfaction of their customers and their employees. Being a good manager and having poor performing and unmotivated employees and dissatisfied customers is a contradiction in terms.

At our place, our best managers get consistently high ratings on their customer satisfaction ratings and on our employees climate assessments. Customers and employees think highly of them because they perform so well on their two principal functions: team building and leadership and service management. Who are the great managers? By their employees' morale and their customers' enthusiasm you will know them. Because employee morale is so closely connected with service excellence and since both are dependent on good management, CQI organizations do all they can to be sure that customers and employees have a good manager.

The most important lessons our department heads learn on team leadership and service management take place during the interactions they have with their own supervisors, the hospital's corporate staff. For better or for worse, slowly, "imperceptibly" but very definitely, managers tend to increasingly become like their bosses. The vice-presidents on the corporate staff provide an excellent example of collaboration and friendship with each other and set the tone for the kind of interdepartmental cooperation necessary to consistently please patients.

For example, I'm not sure I have ever received a formal memo from any of my corporate colleagues in the last ten years. Yet it would be an exceptional day when I don't get or pay a personal visit or get a handwritten note on some item of business to every one of my corporate colleagues. "Here's something we're looking at that affects you. What do you think?" "Such and such happened. I'm letting you know so you don't get blind-sided." "Here's something I came across I thought you might like to read." Anybody at The Williamsport Hospital & Medical Center will tell you that the corporate staff is tight—that they really work together. I'm pleased to say, it's rubbed off on the rest of our management staff.

Through their personal involvement in departmental service planning, through work-a-day-in-my-shoes, through personal participation in CQI tool training and projects, through their own view of themselves as service executives, and through their coaching and evaluation of department heads, the corporate staff daily inculcate into our managers our expectation: They're to build service teams and create a long-term loyal clientele.

Without this corporate modeling, leadership, and cheerleading, all the training in the world wouldn't have much of an effect in the long run. But just as an organization's service culture provides the kind of atmosphere in which CQI methods can flourish, so, too, the daily service and team playing style of the hospital's senior executives provide the kind of environment in which management training can have an enormous positive impact. The human resources department serves as a coach to our corporate staff in their relationships with their department heads. I can't think of a time when any of our vice-presidents— our COO, Steve Johnson, our vice-president of nursing, Jeannie Hill, our assistant vice-president for nursing, Candy Dewar, our vice-president for finance, Mike Scherneck, and the rest of the corporate team— have had a serious personnel problem and did not approach either Dave Heiney, our director of employee relations or me for our input, reactions, and advice. Human resources also provides all the leadership, service management, and customer relations training necessary to support our corporate staff's efforts at ensuring every employee's right to a good manager.

HIRING THE BEST PEOPLE:
The Behavior-Based Model
of Employment and Interviewing

Briefly describe the step by step process you follow in selecting a person for a position you are trying to fill. Okay, you say, the objective is to get the best person for the job. So far, so good. Now jot down exactly what you will do to make sure that will happen. Up until eight years ago, when it came to describing my method for selecting employment candidates, there wasn't much I could say beyond the importance of asking open-ended questions.

There I was with many years in human resources facing this reality: The quality of our service systems and the effectiveness of our healthcare outcomes were largely dependent on the quality of the people who work for us. About 15 percent, or anywhere between 250 and 300 employees leave the hospital every year and approximately that number were hired to fill their places. And I couldn't honestly set about improving the process through which these selections were made, because there was no process. What we did when we hired someone was what everybody I knew did when they hired someone. We did it by the seat of our pants and on a gut feeling. We relied on instincts, made subjective judgments, and then made the best of what we got. That was before I was introduced to Dr. Paul Green's behavior-based model of employment selection, learned it, applied it, and together with my colleagues on the quality council installed it as required practice here at The Williamsport Hospital & Medical Center.

The underlying assumption of the behavior-based model is that past performance, though not infallible, is the best predictor of future performance. A baseball player who has hit .300 or better in each of the last five years of play is more likely to hit at a .300 average in the future than a ball player who has hit under .250 in the past five years. A candidate with demonstrated competence in the skills required for a new open position is more likely to succeed in the new job than a candidate who has not demonstrated competence in those skill areas in his past job performance. The Romans had a great saying that capsulized the wisdom behind this model: *"Ab esse ad posse, valet elatio sed non ab posse ad esse."* We'd probably say, "If you have already done it, you can probably do it again. If you haven't done it before, let us pray."

At The Williamsport Hospital & Medical Center, we have expanded the behavior-based model from its origins as a process of interviewing into a process of employee selection. We have applied the essential methodology to include the processes by which we examine and screen resumés and conduct reference checks and observe performance. The idea is to gain as much information as possible from as many direct or indirect sources of information as possible about the past job-related demonstrated competence of candidates in the high-priority skill areas required by the new job.

181

KICKING THE TIRES BEFORE BUYING THE CAR:
Our Employee Certification Program

Sometimes what you think you see isn't quite what you get. I was in the middle of a heated reprimand to my son, Sean, then 15, as we drove home when I interrupted myself to ask Sean if he was hungry. He said he was; so I pulled into a Wendy's. "What do you want," I asked sharply. "A double cheeseburger." "Double cheese burger," I repeated through the window. "French fries." "French fries," I relayed. "A coke and a chocolate frosty," Sean managed to say before he broke into laughter. "What's so funny?" I demanded. "Look out the window, Dad." Outside the window stood a gigantic, brightly painted garbage container into which I was barking my order. I, too, broke out laughing. "You tell anyone about this," I told him, "and you're going to be terra firmatically impaired."

The same kind of misperception can occur during an interview with a prospective employment candidate. Occasionally, managers hire new employees who turn out to be quite different once they start working than they first appeared to be during the application and interview phases of the employment process. I remember one new employee who impressed her interviewers so much, she was offered a highly sought-after professional position with us. When she went down to get a required test in our laboratory on the day she was hired, she behaved boorishly, offensively and obnoxiously toward four different laboratory employees. After a confab among the hiring department head, our director of laboratory services and our director of employee relations, we decided to terminate the young lady immediately. To my knowledge, hers was the shortest career of any employee in our hospital's 120-year history. We figured that if she was going to be so unC.A.R.E.ing during the start of the honeymoon right after the courtship, she was likely to be unbearable after the marriage was consummated. She may be the only employee we ever had who had a date-of-hire but no first-day-of-work.

Every once in a while, we hire a mismatch for a job; we make hiring mistakes. About a year ago, we installed an employee certification program that keeps these mistakes from being irreparable and interminable. We picked up the idea from Horst Schultz, the COO of the Ritz Carlton, a 1993 Malcolm Baldrige National Quality Award winner.

182

The certification program is simple. Two weeks before the end of our 90-day probation period, a new hire's supervisor must indicate in writing on a standard certification form (see Resource 7-2) that a new employee is: certified as a regular employee in his new position, required to have his probationary period extended for a specified period of time to complete his certification review, or deemed not to have demonstrated the potential to merit certification for the job in any one or more of the three dimensions of quality. A supervisor's department head must sign off on every submitted certification form.

Before the institution of this certification program, probationary periods typically slipped by without any formal indication of the new employee's actual competence except in the very worst of cases. Since we began the certification program, 10 percent of our new hires have had their probationary periods extended for additional training and observation.

We have extended the probationary period of employees for the following kinds of reasons:

- Inadequate fulfillment of the C.A.R.E. behaviors.
- Borderline attainment of performance standards, for example, marginal completion of the cleaning check-out list of patient rooms.
- Barely adequate compliance with attendance and punctuality standards.
- Failure to completely satisfy clinical expectations.
- Performance that indicates satisfaction with the merely passable.

As a general rule, we extend the probationary period for any employee who raises serious concerns that they will not meet our task and relational standards of performance if they are reinstated as certified regular employees.

In addition, though our termination rate for employees during their probationary period remains low, it has doubled since the program started. Before employees went from probationary status to regular status without "The *Good Housekeeping* seal of approval." If the supervisor did nothing, the new employee was in. Now supervisors are being held accountable for the employees they hire by being forced to make a decision about whether to retain the employee. In the long run, we anticipate that this program will reduce the number of culturally antagonistic problem employees. And that's good news for our

Resource 7-2. Sample Managerial Certification Form

MANAGERIAL CERTIFICATION

NAME: _____

DEPARTMENT:_____

DATE: _____

I hereby confirm that during his/her probationary period

_____
(employee's name)

1)   has demonstrated competence in the required skill areas of his/her job duties and responsibilities.

_____ yes   _____ no

2)   exhibits the C.A.R.E. behaviors with *all* fellow employees, patients, visitors, physicians, and other customers.

_____ yes   _____ no

3)   has been taught, understands, and practices those portions of his/her job described in our departmental quality service plan.

_____ yes   _____ no

And, I assert that, having finished his/her 90 day probationary period,

_____
(employee's name)

is _____   is not _____

approved as a(n) _____ subject to
(job title)

regular hospital-mandated performance standards.

Therefore, I recommend that this employee (check the appropriate choice):

- be given the status of a regular employee.
- have his/her probationary period extended for _____.
- be terminated.   (number of days)

_____   _____
Supervisor's signature   Department head signature

Resource 7-2.　Sample Managerial Certification Form
(continued)

Nothing in this managerial certification should be construed as a contract nor should achieving regular status be construed as having permanent employment.
Comments:

_____

_____

_____

_____

_____

_____

Send original to human resources and forward a copy to the division vice-president

---

customers and employees who would otherwise have had to contend with them.

BRINGING OUR EMPLOYEES INTO THE CENTER
OF OUR BUSINESS: Organizational Climate Assessments

When I was on the island of Maui in the state of Hawaii last year, I learned that it takes 2,000 pounds of water to produce one pound of sugar. I added that fact to the other trivia that clutters my mind. It takes up to 40 to 50 tomatoes to yield 8 ounces of dried tomatoes. It takes 17 pounds of saffron flowers to make one $70 ounce of saffron. When you're trying to run an operation that's a cut-above-the-rest you often need to put in a ton of input to get a gram of outcome. In organizational settings, it takes a whole lot of managerial effort over a long period of time to generate the smallest concentration of employee goodwill and trust. Over the last 10 years, our corporate staff, department heads, and supervisors—our entire management team—have watched their gargantuan efforts slowly build, grow, and compound into some astounding payoffs. These results are especially remarkable because they run counter to national trends. Nationwide over the last 20 years, while mandates for total quality have increased, employee trust in management has fallen to all-time lows.

Here are a few examples of the progress our management team has made over the last decade in improving this hospital's organizational climate:

Overall Employee Ratings
1984-1985—69 percent
1993-1994—90 percent
Improvement—30 percent
*Employees are now responding positively to all items

Employees Feel Valued
1984-1985—57 percent
1993-1994—96 percent
Improvement—68 percent
*This item is the most telling and indicative measure of an exemplary corporate culture

Department Head/Supervisor Leadership
1984-1985—64 percent
1993-1994—85 percent
Improvement—32 percent
*Employees responding positively to the eight items affected predominantly by mid-level front-line supervisory leadership

Senior Management Leadership
1984-1985—67 percent
1993-1994—93 percent
Improvement—39 percent
*Employees responding positively to the seven items affected predominantly by the leadership of the senior management staff

The changes brought about by our management staff are phenomenal. Simply maintaining these ratings will be a formidable task.

Periodically, over the past 10 years, we have conducted organizational climate assessments of our employees. We always do it ourselves. So it doesn't cost us anything. We always administer the survey at mandatory events like our annual Quality C.A.R.E. program in order to ensure close to a 100% response rate. We ensure anonymity. We share the results. (Resource 7-3 shows the results from previous climate assessments.) We analyze our data hospital wide and department by department. The final product of our work are hospitalwide and departmental climate improvement plans whose implementation is monitored and evaluated. Slowly but surely, we've watched the numbers eke up to a point that we would all like to sustain and even improve further.

HUMAN RESOURCES DEPARTMENT POLICIES AND PRACTICES: Supporting the Unified Pursuit of CQI

I remain particularly concerned about the responses to several items on our organizational climate assessment. Positive ratings have gone up on all of these items over the last 10 years—but not nearly enough as far as I'm concerned. A couple of these items are:

6. Promotions here are based on qualifications.
   1984-1985 39 percent
   1993-1994 65 percent
15. There are good opportunities to grow and advance here.
    1984-1985 48 percent
    1993-1994 78 percent

There are some strong reasons these items are hard to improve even if the effort is made. On promotions, for example, one can argue that every time a promotion is conferred, one person is happy and a half dozen or more who think they are equally qualified are not so happy. On opportunities to advance, one can say that in many hospital departments, it is very difficult to justify the creation of structures to allow for advancement over time. Then, too, the improvement on these items— intractable as they are—is truly remarkable.

Resource 7-3.   Human Resources Climate Assessment

		Positive Rating		
		1985 (%)	**1991 (%)**	**1994 (%)**	**Change**
1.	Communication from our department head is frank and honest.	58	82	85	27
2.	The corporate staff runs this organization effectively.	65	87	96	31
3.	The work rules and policies in my department make sense.	63	84	87	24
4.	Overall hospital rules and policies make sense.	76	93	96	20
5.	The working conditions in our department are good.	58	78	84	26
6.	Promotions here are based on merit and qualifications.	39	55	69	30
7.	People in different departments cooperate well with each other.	60	76	85	25
8.	Overall, The Williamsport Hospital is a good place to work.	90	97	99	9
9.	My job is interesting and challenging.	89	92	95	6
10.	My supervisor recognizes me when I do a good job.	64	81	83	19
11.	I receive the information I need to do my job properly.	71	86	88	17
12.	Our supervisors are reasonably responsive to employee's needs and concerns.	63	84	83	20
13.	I feel free to discuss problems and concerns with my supervisor.	69	84	83	14
14.	The corporate staff is reasonably responsive to employee's needs and concerns.	61	80	91	30
15.	There are good opportunities to grow and advance here.	48	73	76	28
16.	Most people in our department get along well with each other.	78	85	88	10

Resource 7-3.   Human Resources
Climate Assessment *(continued)*

		Positive Rating		
	1985 (%)	1991 (%)	1994 (%)	Change
17. Generally, The Williamsport Hospital is a safe place to work.	94	99	99	5
18. I feel pleased to work at The Williamsport Hospital & Medical Center.	91	97	98	7
19. I have the tools and equipment to do my job properly.	78	89	94	16
20. The work rules and policies in my department are fairly administered.	67	83	83	16
21. Employees here already have effective ways of bringing their suggestions and ideas to management's attention.	61	84	89	28
22. The Williamsport Hospital responds positively and quickly to customer feedback.	76	90	97	21
23. Employees here are expected to provide the very best in patient care.	97	98	99	2
24. The Williamsport Hospital really values its employees.	57	80	92	35
25. Employees in my department have adequate ways of expressing their views on decisions that affect them.	—	83	85	2
26. I am proud to be an employee of The Williamsport Hospital & Medical Center	—	97	99	2
27. I would not have any reservations about having a member of my family cared for at The Williamsport Hospital & Medical Center.	—	97	99	2
28. I would feel comfortable referring friends, neighbors, and community members to The Williamsport Hospital & Medical Center.	—	98	99	1
29. The Williamsport Hospital & Medical Center is a better place to work than most other area organizations.	—	95	99	4
30. The Williamsport Hospital & Medical Center is the best hospital in the region.	—	95	99	4

Still, I would like us to be creative in finding ways to do better than we have done so far. With regard to promotions, for example, we have very few substantial goodies available to us to give to excellent performers related to ego-status and self-actualization besides advancement. Promotions are strong motivators. We need to find ways to earn our employees' view that we dispense them fairly. With regard to growth opportunities, we believe that organizations tend to grow and to grow successfully the better they get at growing people. People feel motivated to strive for the organization's growth if company success also means personal advancement. The unified pursuit of CQI is substantial at high levels in companies perceived as fair and objective in their promotions and concerned about personal advancement. Consequently, good is not good enough.

Human resources needs to ask the following question about each and every one of its personnel policies and practices: What can we do to increase the likelihood that this policy or practice will get people to do their personal bests together on behalf of the customer? So, for example, we've got to have systems in place ensuring that we:

- Hire the best available talent. We rely heavily on the behavior-based model.
- Discipline fairly and consistently. We require the involvement of our director of employee relations from beginning to end of every case of discipline to ensure uniformity.
- Terminate employees professionally and with sensitivity. Our director of employee relations alone has the final word on a termination and coaches managers throughout the process in cases in which termination is justified. Our vice-president for human resources gives a thorough review to all appealed terminations.

And so, too, on down the line of every policy and practice. Each conveys to our employees how we trust and value them and how seriously we are to be taken when we say that they are our most valuable asset.

THE QUALITY SECRET: Integrating the Human Resources Function With the Hospital's Business Strategy

Don Creamer is fond of saying: "If you have a decision to make and don't know what to do, look at our value statement and you cannot go wrong":

> Continuously demonstrate the highest regard for the two most important groups of people in our institution: our employees and our customers.

Over the years, we have made all of our strategic and service decisions with this value in mind. Ten years ago, we decided to cut costs by reducing full-time equivalents over time without lay-offs: we have reduced our workforce by 10 percent—150 full-time equivalents without a lay-off. We have expanded our services to include open heart surgery and comprehensive care to meet our community's healthcare needs and to ensure better job security for our employees. We opted to employ family practice physicians rather than develop convenient care centers to increase market share that ensures job security. And just this year, among all the business options available to us, we decided to form an alliance with our previous competitors because, among other important reasons, such an alliance would be in the best interest of our employees as well as the community.

Quite often, the job of director of human resources is, in economist Lester Thurow's words, "a specialized, off-at-the-edge-of-the-corporation job." Frequently, the director of human resources does not even get consulted about major strategic decisions. The human resources director is often way down in the corporation's pecking order. In the United States, corporate officers in charge of counting the beans are far more influential and better compensated than the managers (often not a vice-president) who are in charge of those who earn the beans. The reason for this is that they are seen to be more valuable to CEOs than directors of human resources. In this kind of atmosphere, people are just another input to operations to be hired—and more recently the least number at the lowest cost—pretty much the way supplies and equipment are bought. They are not members of the team. Sometimes, they are the enemy.

The turnover rate in American businesses is about 4 percent a month. In Japan, the turnover rate is about 4 percent a year! Misguided hospital managers sometimes think that turnover means lower wages and greater efficiency. They would, for example, rather pay entry-level wages to some support people then pay high wages to long-term employees. These managers understand neither the cost of turnover nor the value of committed employees.

We still haven't learned what the military learned years ago: effective armies need a central cadre of experienced troops. Sure they need some infusion of new blood, but they always need a core of committed, motivated, well-trained soldiers. Some military experts say that the frequent rotation of individuals in Vietnam was one of the big tactical mistakes of the war. Bonding didn't happen because individuals—not platoons and companies—were typically rotated in and out of battle. Armies know that teamwork is more important than individual brilliance. Human resources directors in service industries ought to know that too. Teamwork is necessary for quality, which is necessary for financial success. Human resources directors ought to make that connection known and believed by the organization's decision makers. And they ought to help make the teamwork necessary for quality to happen.

Human resources directors often express the desire to become partners with the hospital's leadership in planning the institutions business strategy. Nevertheless, they and their staffs then go on to define their own human resources mission and goals in ways that are not intimately connected with the organization's mission, purpose, and goals. The human resources goal—employees unified in the pursuit of continuous quality improvement—is not only obviously and directly related to the corporate goal of continuous quality improvement, employees unified in the pursuit of CQI *is* the indispensable prerequisite for successfully achieving the organization's business strategy.

Positive morale is the link to CQI! Positive morale ensures the delivery of quality, and the achievement of quality ensures the maintenance of a positive morale. In hospitals with a vibrant CQI culture, human resources and CQI are inextricably interwoven. As I have said:

People must want to do something before they can do it. Human resources departments that shape and fashion all they do and influence to achieve a workforce united in the pursuit of CQI do not have to request a partnership role in strategic planning. They will, by the very nature of what they contribute, be a valued and welcomed collaborator in the process.

8

Past Outcomes
and Future Expectations

"Yesterday is a canceled check. Today is cash on the line.
Tomorrow is a promissory note."

—Anonymous

A tourist in the nation's capital was riding by a government archives
building in a cab. Carved in stone toward the top of the building were
the words: "Past is Prologue." The puzzled tourist asked the cabby
what that meant. "It means," said the cabby, "you ain't seen nothing
yet."

That's pretty much the attitude of the folks here at The Williamsport Hospital & Medical Center as we prepare to spring out of the starting blocks into our tenth year of CQI. I often repeat this saying to our
employees: There are three kinds of people in this world. People who
make things happen. People who watch things happen. And people
who wonder what the hell happened. We make a special effort to be
people who make rather than merely take our future. We want to
remain an organization that makes things happen.

But much of the recent literature has been filled with tales of CQI
failure. "Hospitals Question the Return on Their TQM Investment"
screams one headline from a recent issue of *Hospitals and Health Networks*. The title of a new book: *Why TQM Fails*. There have been successes and where there have been, the reasons given for success
include: the view of CQI as a long-term investment; perseverance and
patience; the integration of CQI beliefs, goals, and practices into the
culture and daily life of an institution; an effective and committed

leadership group; and the pervasion of CQI operational ideals into other key institutional functions like marketing, strategic planning, internal communications, and the maintenance of an organizational climate conducive to the flourishing of CQI values and dedicated work.

As we begin our tenth year of formally planned quality improvement, we pause to reckon the CQI benefits we have reaped, the opportunities, trends, and obstacles facing our future CQI endeavors and the strategic changes we will make to ensure that our patients and other customers receive the very best well into the next century.

C.A.R.E. OUTCOMES: Nice Guys Finish First

One hundred and thirty years ago, Dr. Richard Orsler said: "It's more important to know what kind of patient has the disease than it is to know what kind of disease the patient has." It's surely at least *just* as important. And when that piece of advice is taken to heart and lived daily, the one thing that counts happens: patients are satisfied. And as Irwin Press argues in "Patient Satisfaction" (*Hospitals and Health Networks,* March 5, 1994): "Satisfied patients will heal better, complain less, be more likely to return and less likely to sue." Dr. Press calls patient satisfaction "the one indicator you can't put a spin on . . . Patients are either satisfied or they're not; no excuse can make a bad experience pleasant. Patients, of course, are the experts at judging the quality of care from the recipient's perspective. Of all outcome indicators, patient satisfaction reflects the broadest range of experience with the entire institution. It encompasses technical interventions, personal interactions, logistical, environmental, dietary, and a host of other experiences with care."

We are elated that our customers and our employees are as satisfied as they are with The Williamsport Hospital & Medical Center. Here are some selected three-year trends that indicate the level of satisfaction experienced by our patients, our employees, and our physicians.

Patient feedback

The only lasting asset a company has is happy customers. Our focus has always been on the subjective perception of customers over the long haul. Here are some key things we know about our customers:

- 99.6 percent would return and recommend us. Virtually all of the 0.4 percent who would not return wouldn't because they live outside the area.
- 57.7 percent indicate they thought our service improved since their last visit
- 41.2 percent say that our service has remained at the same high level of quality they experienced previously
- An independent Gallup poll shows that our hospital enjoyed among the highest patient satisfaction levels recorded in the Mid-Atlantic region: more than 97 percent overall satisfaction rate at versus 93 percent in the other hospitals studied.
- An independent study conducted by the Voluntary Hospitals of America rates our nursing and medical staff in the superior range. In this study, more than 99 percent of our patients said they would return to our hospital compared to 93 percent of patients at other hospitals and 97 percent of our patients said they would recommend us to others compared to 93 percent of patients elsewhere.

Many people are not impressed by numbers. I found that out when I led a study of problem drinking on the nation's railroads between 1978 and 1980. The multimillion dollar study developed a mound of compelling statistics about the enormity and severity of the problem. But congressional subcommittees were moved more by the anecdotal experience of individual alcoholic railroad employees than by the numbers.

Because the concrete tends to make more of an impression than statistics, the following letter may give a flavor to the numbers given above:

Dear Mr. Creamer:

I want to express my complete satisfaction during my recent hospital visit of three days for the efficiency, professionalism, and especially *kindness* and *interest* of *every* member of your staff with whom I came in contact. I find it most unusual to find *every* person so caring. I felt so cared for and safe.

As an R.N., I am especially particular; so I congratulate your facility and thank you for a job well done.

Sincerely,
Fran L. Clausen

In Quality Health Care & Outcomes (July 1993), Avedis Donabedian, M.D., resoundingly echoes Dr. Press's view about patient satisfaction: "To the extent that satisfaction is an aspect of well-being, it may be considered an outcome of care . . . satisfaction or dissatisfaction reflects the patient's judgment on all aspects of care, including the technical process, the interpersonal process, and the outcomes of care, as well as the structural attributes of the settings in which care is provided. Patient satisfaction can also influence the effectiveness of therapy. Satisfied patients are more likely to cooperate with providers, communicate medically important information, comply with treatment, and show an interest in health education."

People make decisions on healthcare largely based on their own personal satisfaction. That's why we will continue to use patient feedback as *the key source* of information to guide our quality work—not merely a source that complements other sources. If we continually achieve the trackable subjective outcome of patient enthusiasm over the long run, it's an odds on bet that we will also earn high marks for better than most for medical outcomes and practices.

Employee satisfaction with service quality

My boss, Don Creamer, often says: "If you've got a good box and a bad product, you'll sell one box of your product. If you have a bad box and a good product, you won't sell a single box. If you've got a good box, a good product, and your employees believe you do, your biggest problem will be maintaining an ample supply." We are gratified to know that our employees consider our hospital a great place to receive healthcare and a great place to work: As noted, our 1993-94 climate assessment shows that:

- 99.8 percent of employees believe the hospital is committed to the highest quality medical care and customer service
- 99.8 percent of employees would recommend our hospital to relatives, friends and acquaintances.
- 93.4 percent of our employees believe that the hospital really values its employees.

We put a great deal of stock in these numbers because we agree with Dr. Press that: ". . . patient satisfaction is more than an indicator.

Its broad significance lies in the fact that it is also a *component* of care. When patients are more satisfied, a host of additional factors makes it impact on care, including enhancement of trust, leading to greater compliance, increased tolerance of uncomfortable or frightening interventions, and increased tolerance of delays."

Medical staff satisfaction

"In ioco veritas," the ancient Romans used to say. "In the joke, lurks the truth" is my free rendition of that quote. In the world of healthcare, the most frequent object of jokes told by hospital administrators, with or without the benefit of alcohol, are physicians. My physician friends tell me not to feel guilty about that fact because in physician circles, it works out the other way too.

Given this backdrop, we are pleased that our physicians have some nice things to say about us. That's important because ever closer collaboration with our medical staff will be an even greater requirement for future success. We are pleased to have a solid basis on which to deepen these relationships. The physician survey we conducted this year indicates that:

- 97 percent of our physicians indicate high levels of satisfaction with our hospital's services.
- A majority of them expect their use of the hospital to increase in the future.
- 93 percent rate hospital-physician communications as effective or very effective.

For more than seven years now, our physicians have participated in a program that honors doctors who are exemplars of C.A.R.E., the first dimension of quality. We have recognized 32 physicians as C.A.R.E. physicians of the month and seven as C.A.R.E. physicians of the year. The executive committee of the medical staff makes the final selections for C.A.R.E. physicians. Physicians are eligible for and often receive magic moments for individual acts of go-beyond service. Every year at our family practice residency graduation, a resident physician is selected as the recipient of the Cap Peter's Memorial Award, a reward named after a young deceased resident and given to a second-year student who best exemplifies caring qualities and shows a high level of respect for his or her peers. Our residents are evaluated on the interpersonal dimension of quality. And the vast majority of family practice physicians in our community are graduates of this program and are employees of The Williamsport Hospital & Medical Center. Physicians participate in our system-focused TQM efforts in three ways. Five physicians serve on our MEDIMPROVE committee, which has oversight responsibility for all projects related to systems improvement. CQI projects use our medical staff as information resources on all system initiatives. About a half dozen work on CQI teams. Finally, all of the teams working on "patient" management guidelines—about 15 right now—have heavy physician involvement.

TQM OUTCOMES: Getting Out the Kinks

We are highly sensitive to dramatically destructive threats and events. At the same time, we are often oblivious to slowly or quietly deteriorating processes. Yet when you think about it, many of the things that go wrong personally, famially, socially, nationally, internationally, and universally (becoming alcoholic, divorce, familial breakdown, the breakdown and aging of our infrastructure, environmental degeneration, the trashing of space) take place slowly over time. So too with our service processes. We stand by as our service systems slowly, gradually get worse and worse and worse.

One of the most important vehicles for ensuring this sort of thing doesn't happen as often as it otherwise would in our place is our quality service plan. As I've explained before, our quality service plan is an annual updated description of each department's most important customers, these customers' key moments of truth in the service cycle, their most important expectations for these moments of truth, the exact sequence of actions or the system that employees are to follow to transform these moments of truth into magic moments. One of our most valuable TQM results is a response system for every moment of truth.

The other principal mechanisms we use are the various kinds of CQI teams described in chapter 5: our cycle of service teams; our departmental CQI teams, our spin-off teams; and our SWAT teams. These teams continue to generate system improvements every year. For example, this year, among the 100 or so quality projects completed were the following randomly chosen measurable improvements:

- Interdepartmental transport committee—reduction in delivery time and increase in service coverage.
- Radiology, lab, billing, family practice, workcenter—more timely, accurate scheduling, results, and points of entry.
- Dietary—patient overall satisfaction with food to 95 percent.
- ER, 4 East, 3 East, ICU, 4 West—patient transfer to room in acceptable time, appropriate report from ER to unit, preparation on unit, increased trust among departments.
- MIS, fiscal services, human resources, nursing—implementation of a time and attendance system and increased accountability.
- ER—reduction in patient departures to another hospital's ER from 70/month to 3/month in 1993.
- Cardiac surgery team—the integration of CQI into program planning (continuous quality visioning)—organized 14 months before the program began.

We have been implementing more than 100 major quality-improvement plans that affect our service systems in each of the last six years. And our patients tell us: It shows.

MEDIMPROVE OUTCOMES: On Feeling Fit and Sassy

When it's all said and done, no one wants to hear: The staff was caring, things ran smoothly, the operation was successful, but the patient died! Positive medical outcomes are harder to demonstrate than subjective patient outcomes. But we work hard at it and have achieved gratifying results like the following:

- Our complication and death rates are 15 percent to 36 percent better than predicted when compared to outcomes measured nationally by the respected MedisGroup Data Base.
- Our complication and death rates are at or below the predicted rates for illnesses analyzed by our state in the Pennsylvania Hospital Effectiveness Report.

- Deaths in our intensive care unit are significantly less than predicted according to the analysis done by our MIS department from information provided by our medical records and our intensive care unit. MIS use a severity of disease classification software package called APACHE (*Acute Physiological Score and Chronic Health Evaluation*) developed for the National Institutes of Health and the Government Accounting Office by William A. Knaus, M.D., Jack E. Zimmerman, M.D., Douglas P. Wagner, Ph.D., and Elizabeth A. Draper, R.N.
- Our infection rates—including nosocomial, surgical, non-specific, respiratory, and central line infections—are well below the averages reported by the Centers for Disease Control.
- Our rehabilitation center has achieved a 25 percent improvement in its treatment outcomes as measured by the Functional Improvement Measurement System (FIMS) and now does better than regional and national averages.

To maintain the medical and clinical quality exemplified in these areas, we do a lot of work on defining the best practices, or in the words of the trade, clinical pathways—the ways to handle cases and do procedures that are most likely to have a positive outcome. Among the approximately 25 MEDIMPROVE projects now in progress are the following areas of opportunity:

- *Inpatient chemotherapy:*
  —Streamline process for administration of oncologies.
  —Reduce length of stay.
  —Increase patient satisfaction.
  —Establish a clinical pathway.
- *Psychiatric unit: initial assessment for major depression:*
  —Eliminate duplication of assessment.
  —Develop clinical pathway.
  —Reduce length of stay.
- *Cerebral vascular accident/stroke:*
  —Develop practice guidelines for pre-hospital care, first through third days of stay and fourth day through discharge.
- *Pre-admission testing/A.M. admission for same-day surgery:*
  —Integration of service delivery to reduce waiting times, improve result reporting, the admission process, and patient satisfaction.

- *Angioplasty:*
  —a continuous visioning opportunity.
  —prospective application of CQI principles to the new angioplasty service well in advance of its start date.
- *Top-ten surgeries:*
  —together with select surgeons, establish best practice guidelines for most frequent inpatient surgical patients.
- *Major joint procedures:*
  —design a multidisciplinary approval to develop best practice guidelines for patients undergoing major joint procedures.

Our most exciting MEDIMPROVE result for this year: a five-year plan to develop practice guidelines on selected case types based on volumes, cost, and difficulty.

BUSINESS OUTCOMES: So What's the Bottom Line?

You can't have a mission without a margin, CEOs are fond of saying. One thing about truisms—they're usually true. Most CEOs can readily identify with Charles J. Givens, author of *Wealth Without Risk* (Simon & Schuster, 1991), when he said: "When it comes to your company's money, you are one of two things—a victor or a victim," a winner or a loser. As every entrepreneur knows, the right to do business must be earned not assumed. CEOs have the scary responsibility of making the bottom line black after what's going out has been subtracted from what's coming in. No wonder, then, that CEOs need to be assured that quality makes dollars and cents as well as sense.

Our 10 years of CQI corroborates the basic finding of the profit impact measurement studies (PIMS): quality is good business. Here are some examples of business results we enjoyed because of CQI:

- Average cost per discharge at The Williamsport Hospital & Medical Center—$4,725 versus $5,550 (state average) versus $5,648 (regional average) versus $6,079 (national average).
- Average charge per discharge at The Williamsport Hospital & Medical Center—$5,014 versus $8,074 (state average)
- Open heart surgery charges at The Williamsport Hospital & Medical Center—$26,000 versus $50,150 (state average) versus $23,658 (state low) versus $101,716 (state high).

- $3.6M in savings from product and supply standardization committee analysis of more than 200 items and related systems in the past eight years.
- Our rehabilitation center, the Gibson Rehabilitation Center of The Williamsport Hospital & Medical Center has increased admissions by 36 percent in the last two years.
- Our occupational health program has entered contractual partnerships with more than 100 business partners in the last two years.
- Our sports medicine program has contractual partnerships with every school district and college in our area.

And finally, profitability. There's one person at every hospital whose job it is, after all the income is received and all the bills are paid—to be sure there is an excess of income over expenses. At The Williamsport Hospital & Medical Center that person is Don Creamer, our CEO and my boss. So I asked him:

- *What are the board's profitability goals?*
  Although The Williamsport Hospital & Medical Center is a not-for-profit organization, the board of managers, nonetheless, recognizes its responsibility to ensure the future of the hospital and its ability to continue to meet the needs of those patients we serve and therefore, the board has maintained an expectation to produce a small operating margin (i.e., bottom-line). Generally, our objective has been an operating margin of approximately 2 percent. The board believes that the responsibility of the hospital remains the provision of high-quality, cost-effective patient services (i.e., value) and therefore, our operating margin goals have been modest and designed only to ensure the opportunity for the provision of new programs and services and the support of overall system objectives.
- *How do we compare with financial performance of other hospitals?*
  We compare ourselves to hospitals in our region and on a national basis of similar size, service, and program. Consistently, the hospital's performance has been between 1.25 and 1.5 times the operating margin of comparable institutions on a regional and a national basis.

- *What do you see as the connection between profitability and quality at The Williamsport Hospital & Medical Center?*
  We believe that there is not simply a connection between our ability to meet operating margin objectives and the hospital's commitment to its quality program, but in fact, an inextricable link between quality and a successful operating margin. The quality program has directly affected the hospital's market share and, therefore, fixed costs, which represent approximately 80 percent of total hospital costs, have been spread over increased numbers of patients, lowering the average cost to all patients and ensuring profitability while producing value for the purchasers of our services. The hospital's market share has increased by nearly 30 percent since the inception of the quality program. There is absolutely no question that our financial success is a direct result of our quality efforts.

Implicit in Don Creamer's explanation of the connection between profitability and quality is an insightful redefinition of organizational success. Profit is obviously an important success factor, but a more balanced view of a hospital's success includes factors like enthusiastically motivated and loyal employees, satisfied patients, and a proud community. Robert Hall argues for this kind of expanded definition of success in *The Soul of the Enterprise: Creating a Dynamic Vision for American Manufacturing* (Oliver Wright, 1993). We at The Williamsport Hospital & Medical Center have long believed what John Naisbitt, the author of *Megatrends* said recently about success in the July 1994 issue of *Total Quality:* "Happy workers—not technology or specific management tools—are the keys to competitive success . . . As technology and other strategic tools become easier to acquire, worker-friendly employees will out perform their more profit-minded competitors by growing margins."

9

Making Three Quality Hospitals a Quality System

"The first step toward creating an improved future is
developing the ability to envision it."

—Anonymous

"It's about time. They should have done it a long time ago." That was
the reaction of most people in Williamsport area when they heard that
three local hospitals were going to consolidate services, coordinate
programs, and unify management—from a strictly operational point of
view, to merge. For decades, The Williamsport Hospital & Medical
Center, Divine Providence Hospital two miles away and Muncy Valley
Hospital 15 miles from Williamsport were intense competitors. All
three of the hospitals had their own emergency rooms, pre-hospital services, pediatric and obstetrical departments, and medical surgical units.
The Williamsport Hospital & Medical Center and Divine Providence
Hospital each had their own heart and lung service, rehabilitation ser-
vices, mental health and psychology services, cancer services, and
MRI units.

In 1992, Divine Providence Hospital bought Muncy Valley Hospital. The primary service area had 6 licensed beds per 1,000 people at a
time when some healthcare futurists predicted the need for as few as
two beds per 100 people. Services, programs, equipment and staff were
still duplicated and largely uncoordinated. Things were just about the
way they still are most places in the country. And Adam Smith and the
supply siders notwithstanding, competition was not lowering costs. It

was having the opposite effect. Enter the consumer and third-party pay-ors who were saying loud and clear: "Keep quality high. Get prices low. We want value."

Value—The Customer's Highest Priority, Reconfiguration of Services—the Organization's High-Focused Response

In July, 1994, our customers had their way. Old competitors have become allies. The Williamsport Hospital & Medical Center and the Providence Health System will serve the communities in their service area as the Susquehanna Healthcare System (SHS). Don Creamer of The Williamsport Hospital & Medical Center, Sister Jean Mohl, president, and Kirby O. Smith, executive vice-president and COO of the Providence Health System came to believe that coming together was the right thing to do for our patients, for our community, for our employees, and for our payors. If it wasn't a vision, that conviction was at least a paradigm smasher. The three of them developed the alliance concept in its rudimentary form and eventually rallied their respective boards, medical staffs, employees, the business community, and the community at large to support these 6 objectives.

- Coordinate the delivery of healthcare services.
- Reduce the cost of healthcare for our region.
- Enhance the quality of care.
- Better serve all elements of the community.
- Improve the health status of the region through health promotion and education.
- Participate in and promote sound health policy.

Over the course of one full year, Don, Sister Jean, and Kirby led the boards and corporate staffs of both institutions through the long painstaking ticklish process of anti-trust review by the Department of Justice at the federal level, and the Attorney General's office in Harrisburg, Pennsylvania. The alliance went forward under the constraints of a legally binding consent decree that mandates $40 million in net savings over the next five years. A put-up-or-shut-up clause of the decree requires the Alliance to cough up anything less than $40 million of savings in cash in 1999 to be used to deliver anything in the form of health services the alliance promised but failed to deliver. The charge and the promise were clearly higher quality and reduced rates of growth in cost—*value.*

The SHS has defined the following mission, value, and vision ⌣ statements as coordinates on their unified value journey:

Mission Statement:
To improve the health status
of the communities we serve
through high-quality,
compassionate, accessible
and cost-effective care.

Value Statement:
What matters most to us are:
Those who receive our care
and
those who provide our care.

Vision Statement:
Be the healthiest community
in the United States.

Under the leadership of Don Creamer, Sister Jean Mohl, and Kirby Smith, board and corporate leaders agreed on a preliminary reconfiguration of services. The medical staffs and management teams of The Williamsport Hospital & Medical Center, Divine Providence Hospital, and Muncy Valley Hospital provided input and refinements to the reconfiguration model. Fourteen work teams developed strategic guidelines for implementing the new model. As a result of all of this work, the service model was reengineered from its pre-SHS form to its post-SHS metamorphosis. (see Resource 9-1)

In general, centers of excellence will be located where long-established preeminence previously existed. The Williamsport Hospital & Medical Center will, for example, retain heart and lung services, including open heart surgery as well as comprehensive rehabilitation. Divine Providence Hospital will house centers of excellence for comprehensive cancer treatment, mental health, and kidney dialysis. Muncy Valley Hospital will feature services for eye treatments. The

Resource 9-1.   The SHS Service Model

Susquehanna Healthcare System		
TWH&MC	**DPH**	**MVH**
Cardiology (invasive)		
Vascular Surgery	Vascular Surgery	
Cardiac Rehab		
Cardiac Surgery		
Cardiac Support (EKGs & Stress Testing)	Cardiac Support (EKGs & Stress Testing)	Cardiac Support (EKGs & Stress Testing)
	Sleep Disorder Lab	
Pulmonary	Pulmonary	Pulmonary
Orthopedic Surgery (Elective/Emergency)	Orthopedic Surgery (Emergency)	Orthopedic Surgery (Elective/ Emergency)
Occupational Medicine		
Neurosurgery (Elective/Emergency)	Neurosurgery (Elective/Emergency)	
Neurology-EEGs	Neurology-EEGs	
Sports Medicine		
Rehab Medicine	Rehab Medicine	Rehab Medicine
Rheumatology	Rheumatology	Rheumatology
	Oncological Surgery	
	Medical Oncology	
	Radiation Oncology	
Urological Surgery	Urological Surgery	Urological Surgery
Gastroenterology	Gastroenterology	Gastroenterology
ENT/Audiology	ENT/Audiology	ENT/Audiology
GYN/Surgery	GYN/Surgery	GYN/Surgery
Women's Center	Women's Center/ Breast Clinic	

Resource 9-1. The SHS Service Model *(continued)*

Susquehanna Healthcare System		
TWH&MC	**DPH**	**MVH**
	Chronic Pain Management	
General Surgery	General Surgery	General Surgery
Anesthesia	Anesthesia	Anesthesia
		Dental-Oral
		Podiatry
Plastic Surgery	Plastic Surgery	
	Ophthalmology/Retinal	Ophthalmology
Emergency Room (24 hr.)	Urgent Care (16 hr.)	Emergency Room (24 hr.)
Prehospital	Prehospital	Prehospital
	Dialysis-Chronic	
Dialysis-Inpatient Acute	Dialysis-Inpatient Acute	
Endocrinology (Diabetes Education)	Endocrinology (Diabetes Education)	Endocrinology (Diabetes Education)
Behavioral Medicine (Psychology)	Behavioral Medicine (Psychiatry/Psychology)	
		Long-Term Care
	Home Health/Hospice	
Obstetrics		
Pediatrics		
General Medicine	General Medicine	General Medicine
Infectious Disease	Infectious Disease	Infectious Disease
Nuclear Medicine	Nuclear Medicine	Nuclear Medicine
Radiology (Special Procedures)	Radiology (MRI)	Radiology

Shaded box indicates not a full-service department.

number of full-service departments will be reduced. Talent will be pooled. Duplication, reduced'or eliminated. The alliance's goal is to do better with less over time. The yardstick is $40 million savings over five years. I'm taking bets we'll do it.

THE SHS TRANSITION WORK GROUPS:
Focus on Continuous Value Improvement

Under the aegis of a group called the alliance transition task force (the alliance's CEO, COO, and selected board members), a steering committee called the alliance core group (selected corporate staff from both systems) established nine working groups to flesh out the strategic reconfiguration plan into a detailed operational plan. With some guidance from a consulting firm, the groups detailed in Resources 9-2 and 9-3 began their work.

The core group instructed these work groups to function as Continuous Value Improvement (CVI) groups in two senses. First they were to make sure that their recommendations would eventually result in continuous value improvement. They were not to simply come up with ideas that would promote quality without regard to cost. At the same time, they were not to cut costs without regard to quality. Quality improvement and cost reduction were to be considered companion, not antithetical, terms. Well-targeted and planned quality improvements often can and do reduce costs. Second, the core group directed the work groups to integrate and apply the CQI process and tools to the planning process, to function as Continuous Visioning Improvement groups (see Resource 9-4).

As the anti-trust analysis proceeded, these groups began to do their work. The groups were not without their false starts and the typical problems experienced by groups at different stages of their activity. Work group participation amounted to a second job. In the end, they came up with transition plans that met the more than $40 million cost reduction target and unquestionably will result in higher-quality services for our community. In some cases, the work groups suggested system refinements; in others, whole-scale radical replacement—in the current jargon reinvention and reengineering. Core group members were astounded at the first-rate job each and every work group achieved. Virtually every recommendation was approved. The price

Resource 9-2.   Work Group Process

Purpose	Process	Outcome
■ Develop a common understanding of operations of DPH, MVH, and TWHMC ■ Begin to identify major differences in philosophy and practice	Identify current practices at DPH, MVH, and TWHMC: • complete worksheets • discuss and highlight differences	■ Comparison of current practices with differences noted ■ Relationships established between employees of both entities
■ Focus work group efforts on opportunities that will result in desired level of integration	Determine priorities for consolidation: • day 1 of new entity • within 6–12 months • within 1–2 years • not in foreseeable future	■ Prioritized list of practices to integrate
■ Identify objective information to support recommendations	Collect additional data as needed	■ Additional rationale for recommendations
■ Identify opportunities for integration	Develop recommendations for integration based on: • service configuration • impact Include potential timing and responsibility	■ Summary of integration opportunities including resource impact, timing and responsibility for implementation
■ Develop an action plan for implementation of recommendations	Create a work plan to implement integration recommendations including: • activity • timing • responsibility • potential implementation issues	■ Implementation plan

213

Resource 9-3. Susquehanna Health System Operational Plan

Work Group	Operational Focus
NURSING/CLINICAL	• General nursing • Operating room, recovery room • Emergency room and paramedics
ANCILLARY	• Lab • Radiology • Cardiopulmonary therapy • Pharmacy • Respiratory therapy • Physical and occupational therapy • Other
INFORMATION TECHNOLOGY	• Telephone/paging • Information Systems
OUTREACH ACTIVITIES	• Home health • Durable medical equipment • Marketing, communication, health ed/promotion • Physician practices
FINANCIAL FUNCTIONS	• Financial reporting • Chart of accounts and general ledger • Patient accounting • Payroll • Risk management • Accounts payable • Medical records
HUMAN RESOURCES	• Compensation/Classification Systems • Employee benefits • Education/training • Employment transition • Policies and procedures
SUPPORT	• Dietary • Maintenance and biomedical engineering • Laundry • Housekeeping • Security • Materials management
MISSION	• The alliance's mission and value statements
CQI	• The alliance's quality business strategy

Resource 9-4.   Service Reconfiguration Implementation Guidelines

---

Work group recommendations have been approved subject to implementation planning and final review and approval by the SHS corporate staff.

Steps to be followed in preparing for and conducting a specific service implementation:

1. Review service configuration schedule with physician SHS liaison committee.

2. Assign implementation management process to the hospital chief operating officer of the facility where service is to be consolidated.

3. The appropriate SHS corporate officer develops a schedule/sequence detailing major support activities needing to be accomplished to support the schedule/sequence and presents to the SHS corporate staff for review and approval.

4. Select and present to the SHS corporate staff, the names of the full implementation team including the following: Product line or function vice-president, affected physicians, managing directors and supervisors, selected employees from human resources and support services, and other personnel as needed. (NOTE: Steps 3 and 4 may be completed simultaneously.)

5. Assigned SHS corporate officer briefs the implementation team using the format/guideline approximately 120 days prior to implementation.

6. Select and announce the new department head using SHS policy approximately 100 days prior to implementation.

7. Implementation team conducts planning.

8. Implementation team briefs SHS chief operating officer and assigned SHS corporate officers approximately 90 days before implementation.

9. SHS corporate officer and selected implementation team members brief SHS corporate staff and chief executive officer on details of the implementation plan using the attached guidelines approximately 85 days prior to implementation.

Resource 9-4. **Service Reconfiguration Implementation Guidelines** *(continued)*

---

10. SHS chief executive officer reviews implementation plan with SHS board and authorizes same approximately 80 days before implementation.

11. Human resources implements personnel selection, reassignment, training, and employee support group program approximately 75 days prior to implementation.

12. Implementation team continues to refine plan up to day of implementation.

13. Marketing and community relations develops community announcement and education plan approximately 60 days prior to implementation.

14. SHS corporate operations team provides ongoing supervision up to and through implementation.

---

work group members paid to get us to this point was summarized most accurately on a coffee cup we gave each member at a party for all of them: I Survived a Work Group!

IMPLEMENTATION PLANNING TEAMS:
Thinking Through the Service Operation Model

Once the SHS corporate staff and the SHS board approved the work groups' recommendations and the reconfiguration of services, the corporate staff invited managers and physicians affected by the reconfiguration to form advisory implementation planning teams. The corporate staff charged these implementation teams with the responsibility of working out details for implementing approved recommendations and for identifying issues, obstacles, and potential problems in effecting the service configuration plan. The corporate staff selected a facilitator for each team and developed and explained the guidelines under which the teams were to operate.

Long before the SHS start date, hospital leaders had encouraged the creation of a physician SHS liaison committee to exchange information and ideas about the reconfiguration model with the senior management of the SHS. The Physician SHS Liaison Committee continues to provide input and feedback to the SHS corporate staff and the work of the implementation teams. Many of the members of these teams—managers and physicians—stand to be personally and professionally affected in varying degrees by the changes that are taking place. The resulting anxieties and concerns understandably render the teams' important work difficult to bring to a successful conclusion. More than ever before, we thought our managers and physicians needed to be sensitive to each other's perspectives and to have a better understanding of the cultural differences between physicians and hospital managers. We found Stephen Shortell's summary of these differences a useful tool in training our facilitators to conduct the discussions of these joint physician-manager teams (see Resource 9-5).

JUST-IN-TIME ALLIANCE TRAINING:
Jump-Starting the Consolidation Process

As the implementation team schedules were being developed, we concluded that our implementation team members and our managers all needed four capabilities to do their work:

- The ability to manage their projects in a common, consistent manner so that each team's work could be integrated with the planning of implementation teams and with those developing facility, MIS, and human resources plans.
- The ability to convey unwelcome news and to respond in a constructive way to the reactions of those who did not receive it well.
- The ability to handle the personal and professional aspects of experiencing a consolidation of services for those required to move to another facility and for those receiving new associates to their department or unit.
- The ability to respond to the survivors and the displaced through a competent and caring application of the alliance's transition plan.

Resource 9-5. Fundamental Cultural Differences Between Health Care Executives and Physicians

Attribute	Health Care Executives	Physicians
Basis of knowledge	Primarily social and management sciences	Primarily biomedical sciences
Exposure to relevant others while in training	Relatively little exposure to physicians, nurses, other health care professionals, or patients	Great deal of exposure to nurses, other healthcare professionals, and patients; little exposure to broader business/economic world of healthcare
Patient focus	Broad: all patients in the organization and the larger community	Narrow: one's individual patients
Time fame of action	Middle to long run; emphasis on positioning the organization for the future	Generally short run; meet immediate needs of patients
Rules of evidence	Understand the need to act on soft qualitative information; loose-linked cause-effect relationships that may not be well understood	Soft qualitative information viewed with skepticism; prefer hard facts; tightly linked cause-effect relationships that are well understood
View of resources	Always limited; challenge lies in allocating scarce resources efficiently and effectively	Resources essentially unlimited or at least should be unlimited; resources should be available to maximize the quality of care
Professional identity	Less cohesive; less well developed	More cohesive; highly developed

SOURCE: Stephen M. Shortell, Ph.D.; *Effective Hospital-Physician Relationships.*

In response to these four sets of needs, we developed and delivered the following training programs with the following objectives for the following participant groups:

1. "Project Management & Scheduling: Helping Noah Build His Ark" developed in-house and based largely on *Effective Project Planning and Management* by W. Alan Randolph and Berry V. Posner (Prentice Hall, 1988).

   Audience: Facilitators of implementation teams and the alliance corporate staff

   Trainers: Tim Schoner, management engineer, Providence Systems and Bob Ireland, management engineering, The Williamsport Hospital & Medical Center

   Objectives:
   - To identify the basic rules for managing projects.
   - To learn how to establish basic project milestones, activities, relationships, and time estimates.
   - To learn how to construct and interpret a project schedule using a Gantt chart.
   - To understand an activity network and critical path method.
   - To use the critical path method and Gantt Charts to communicate project status.

2. "Notifier Training: Remaining Alive After Delivering Bad News" based on a training program developed by Right Associates, a recruitment firm from Norristown, Pennsylvania.

   Audience: Managers and supervisors

   Trainer: Victoria Carper, Wright Associates

   Objectives:
   - To communicate bad news clearly, quickly, and calmly.
   - To be sensitive to employees' feelings while remaining unwavering on the message.
   - To focus employee away from the past and toward the future.

3. "Consolidation Training: Rolling Out the Red Carpet" developed in-house.

Audience: Managers of consolidating departments and units

Trainers: Team led by Sister Joanne Bednars, vice-president for mission, Providence Systems.

Objectives:
- Identify the needs of staff coming to and working at programs consolidated on a particular campus.
- Develop welcoming, orientation, and retention strategies, initiatives, programs, and practices in newly consolidated programs and units.
- Identify and use support resources throughout the system to facilitate a smooth transition.

4. "The Successful Transition Plan: Getting Everyone to Land on Their Feet"

Audience: Human resource managers

Team: Joint human resources team

Objectives:
- Achieve budgeted labor savings of $22 M over five years.
- Assist displaced employees to land comparable positions within or outside the alliance.
- Avoid lay-offs.

All these programs were completed before we ran our unification training for all alliance employees and management leadership training for all managers and supervisors between September 20 and December 15, 1994.

THE SHS FIRST SWAT TEAM:
Transforming the Captive Patient

It's the middle of August. A lot of people are on vacation. The CQI steering committee isn't scheduled to meet until September. And not too long from now, our SHS staff will be encountering their first group of captive patients. Captive patients are patients who have become accustomed to receiving their services at one of the hospitals in the SHS but who, because services have been consolidated at one of the other former competing hospitals, will have to go elsewhere. Talk about the heat generated by the national debate over employee mandates. You ought to talk to someone in our community who has received an admission mandate. Now we're talking choice and people are not happy about having none.

So even before the first meeting of the SHS CQI steering committee, our rotating chairmen, Anthony Deobil and Steve Johnson are instituting a systemwide captive patient CQI SWAT team. Their charge will be to identify captive patients before admission, come up with a system for informing staff who will care for them about their identity and disposition, and devise methods, including training, to gradually transform them from reluctant prisoners into enthusiastic guests. A tall order, that.

The first two services to be consolidated are Pediatrics/Obstetrics-Gynecology and Comprehensive Cancer Services. The first group of patients is going to have to include would-be-patients who, together with their forbearers for as long as anyone can remember, have brought their children into the world at Divine Providence Hospital or Muncy Valley Hospital. Now they will have to come to The Williamsport Hospital & Medical Center. Others suffering from cancer have established long and deep relationships with the staff at Muncy Valley Hospital and at The Williamsport Hospital & Medical Center. Now they will have to go to Divine Providence Hospital. We'll be tracking the satisfaction surveys of our captive patients very closely and will do whatever it takes over time to make them feel comfortable, cared-for, and at home at whichever hospital we're privileged to serve them in.

TAKING CQI SYSTEMWIDE:
Organizational Structures to Support Quality Service

Chapter 1 describes the way The Williamsport Hospital & Medical Center organized itself to make quality service its strategic business objective. The core group assigned CQI leaders from the Providence

Health System and The Williamsport Hospital & Medical Center to a CQI work group to make continuous value improvement the strategic business objective of the SHS. The CQI group defined the alliance's CQI charter, its organizational structure and the roles to be played by everyone in the alliance to achieve the alliance's business objectives.

The CQI Work Group "Quality Charter" for SHS:

Continuous quality improvement is the universally embraced driving force of the Susquehanna Health System and is implemented through the ongoing assessment, improvement, and delivery of high-quality, cost-effective healthcare, service systems, and personal service that not only meet but exceed our customers' expectations.

Notice that this quality charter includes the following elements:

- CQI is the required way of doing business.
- CQI is everyone's job.
- The customer is the final arbiter of quality.
- There are three dimensions to healthcare quality: an outcome dimension, a systems dimension, and a personal service dimension.

Next, the CQI committee defined the CQI structure of the alliance. It is provided in Resource 9-6.

Finally, the CQI work group defined all of the roles within this CQI structure:

- Customer—The customers define quality in terms of their needs and expectations.
- Board of directors (SHS)—The board of directors serves as the steward of the community ultimately responsible for fulfilling the SHS's mission and through their fiduciary role, providing value in the healthcare services.
- CEO—The CEO is the officer of the SHS, vested by the board of directors, with the authority to lead the corporate quality council in developing the quality improvement goals.
- Corporate quality council—The corporate staff serves as the SHS quality council and is accountable to the CEO and customers for establishing and operationalizing the SHS's strategic quality objectives.

Resource 9-6. The SHS CQI Structure

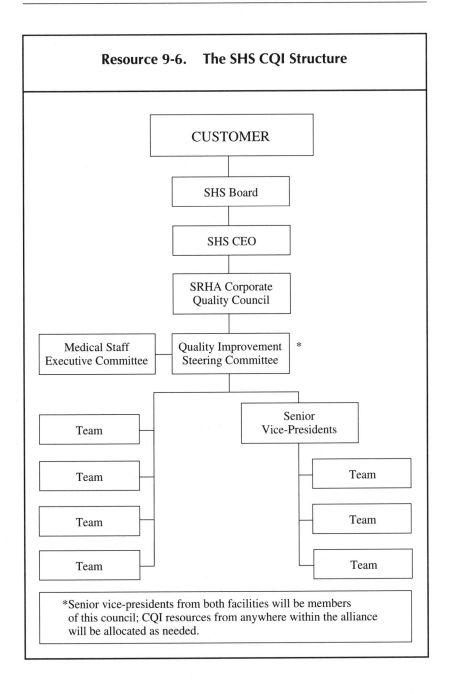

CUSTOMER

SHS Board

SHS CEO

SRHA Corporate
Quality Council

Medical Staff
Executive Committee

Quality Improvement
Steering Committee   *

Senior
Vice-Presidents

Team

Team

Team

Team

Team

Team

Team

Team

*Senior vice-presidents from both facilities will be members
of this council; CQI resources from anywhere within the alliance
will be allocated as needed.

- Quality improvement steering council—The quality improvement steering council establishes and coordinates the SHS's quality strategies. These strategies are accomplished through:
  —Developing the SHS's quality strategic plan.
  —Prioritizing strategies.
  —Initiating teams.
  —Allocating appropriate resources.
  —Communicating outcomes to appropriate bodies.
  —Measuring organizational performance.
- Team:—A team is appointed by the quality improvement council or senior vice-president/president with a defined scope and time table.
- Medical staff executive committee:—Through representation and participation on the quality improvement steering council, the president and president-elect of the medical staffs or their designees will perform the following:
  —Assist in prioritizing strategies.
  —Coordinate the medical staffs for all CQI efforts.
  —Communicate CQI information to the different chairs and departments.
  —Foster participation in and assign medical staff to teams.
  —Assist in and support the implementation of the team action plans.
  —Senior vice-president/president:—The senior vice-president/ president of each hospital is responsible and accountable for operationalizing the CQI process at their facilities and will serve as the chairperson of the quality improvement steering council on an annual rotating basis as an ex-officio member.
  —Quality assurance department—Assuming consolidation of Divine Providence Hospital and The Williamsport Hospital & Medical Center medical staffs, the quality assurance departments and MedisGroup databases should be combined into one department.

At this point in their work, the CQI work group decided to hand on the quality baton to the new SHS corporate staff. The corporate staff will activate the quality improvement steering council, which will, under the corporate staff's leadership, plan and execute the alliance's quality initiatives.

DEVELOPING A WANT-TO WORKFORCE:
Holding Managers Accountable for Employee Morale

Between September and the end of December 1994, we conducted management development and employee training programs for the system's entire management and employee group. In July 1994, we had conducted personal needs assessments with our managers and employees to determine the exact content of the training. We developed specially targeted training for managers and employees in consolidated units. In August 1994, we designed the training. In the next four months, we delivered the training. During that same time, we planned follow-up training for the remainder of the year and beyond.

Some returns are in. We have already conducted an organizational climate assessment among all of SHS employees on The Williamsport Hospital & Medical Center, Divine Providence, and Muncy Valley campuses. During the very first month of the alliance's existence, the alliance corporate staff set system and campus climate assessment goals for the next year. Immediately afterward, human resources staff met with department heads throughout the alliance to set item-by-item and overall climate assessment goals for their individual departments. Next year, before departmental evaluations are done, we will do another systemwide organizational climate assessment. We will evaluate our corporate officers and department heads in part on the difference between next year's and this year's results.

COST-CUTTING STRATEGIES:
From Managing Costs and Use to Reducing Demand

You'll notice that the SHS's mission statement begins with the words "To improve the healthcare status of the communities we serve . . ." and that the SHS's vision statement is "becoming the healthiest community in the country." There's good reason for that.

If you could wave a magic wand and overnight reduce paper work in healthcare by 95 percent, drastically reform the nation's tort system, mandate employer or individual payment for health insurance, make health insurance portable, and eliminate ineligibility based on pre-existing conditions, you wouldn't do much to reduce the cost of healthcare costs as a percentage of our gross domestic product. At least over the short term (who knows about the long term), the only way to contain healthcare costs is to reduce the amount of service provided. The only way to reduce the amount of services provided is to reduce the need for services. That means prevention.

Until now, hospitals and other healthcare providers have been good at making sick people better. That's no mean task and it's no idle boast to say that we in America do it better than anyone else in the world. In the past, we've tried to reduce costs in many ways: preadmission certification, second opinions, Medicare and Medicaid ceilings on the treatment of designated diagnoses, the publication of hospital charges, negotiated volume discounts of one kind or another, delays and reductions in governmentally promised payments and price controls on physician fees for the indigent and the aging. We've tried to reduce the use of services by making individuals pay more out of pocket for healthcare through higher deductibles, larger co-payments, and individual contributions toward healthcare premiums. The result: costs continue to grow per capita, as a percentage of our federal budget and as a percentage of gross domestic product. The national bottom line? Red.

The cure being proposed for this financial mess is prevention. The airwaves are filled with slogans like: "You can only cure retail. You can prevent wholesale." Aside from the question of whether prevention reduces or simply postpones higher healthcare costs, healthcare providers are facing a new challenge in the emphasis on prevention and health maintenance. Our old job used to be making people well. The old measures of quality were recovery, morbidity, and mortality rates. Our new job is keeping people well as well as making people well. The new measures of our alliance will be related to the improved healthcare status in the community. We will be talking about efficient and effective healthcare that maintains health, prevents illness and injury, and appropriately treats disease and injury. We will be looking at new quality indicators like:

- Immunization rates.
- Percent of population with acceptable cholesterol readings.
- Percentage of women receiving prenatal care in the first trimester of pregnancy.

- The functional status of patients six months post-cardiac artery bypass graft.
- Percentage of covered population who visited a healthcare provider within previous two years.

The language we have used at The Williamsport Hospital & Medical Center reveals our recovery orientation and that of the American health system at large. We call the interpersonal dimension of quality: C.A.R.E.; the system dimension, TQM; and revealingly the outcome dimension, *MEDIMPROVE.* One of the most important customers, our payors are changing our business. They want price relief. They think the only concept that has any chance of delivering on this strongly expressed requirement is prevention. In the jargon of The Williamsport Hospital & Medical Center, we will soon have to move from MEDIMPROVE to a term that includes both recovery and prevention—for now let's say HEALTHIMPROVE.

Make no mistake about it, the very purpose and primary goals of the SHS have already been transformed and enlarged by consumers and payors to include an unprecedented emphasis on health maintenance. Those of us who used to be auto mechanics are now being asked to build and maintain cars with a longer life and fewer breakdowns. The quality stars of the past won't necessarily be the quality stars of the future. The language and implementation of these ideas are old but until fairly recently limited. Soon, prevention will be the ball game because of the way health providers will be paid: on a capitated basis (which is discussed later in this chapter).

MANAGED CARE: From a Blank Check
Through the Money Order to Season Tickets

I always tell people: "If you want to enter into a successful new career, watch what I do and then do the opposite." You see, when I was in the fifth grade at St. Peter's Parochial School in Mt. Carmel, Pennsylvania, the fifth-grade boys had to clean the commodes and urinals in the boys' lavatory. Honest! When I entered the sixth grade, the sisters changed the policy. The *sixth*-grade boys had to clean the commodes and urinals in the boys' lavatory. To make a long story short, that critical and trau-matic transition provided me with a predetermined model that has marked my entire career.

In 1982, when I started working in hospitals, I thought I was about to break the pattern. Even I could be a smashing success at running a hospital, I thought. Here's the way things worked. People came to the hospital. No matter how long they stayed, no matter what and how much we did for them, somebody would pay the entire freight. They even had a fancy name for it. They called it retroactive reimbursement. Customers essentially gave you a blank check. Wow! Would I ever be good at filling in the numbers!

I should have known better. It was too good to be true. On July 1, 1984 (a day, which for all hospital administrators is considered a day of infamy against which December 7, 1941 pales by contrast), beginning with the federal government's Medicare program, the era of the blank check ended. Now, hospitals became like delis. "Pastrami with cheese: $3.95. Toppings: $.50 extra." "Appendectomies: $3,000. With compli-cations: $500 extra." So if you were a Medicare patient, came to the emergency room with a heart attack, the hospital was going to get $4,500 for you, period. After examining you, the physician decides you need the drug TPA to break up your clot. TPA costs $2,200 a shot. The hospital has $2,300 left to take care of you. Four days into your stay, the money's gone. You stay three more days. The hospital has to assume the cost for the last three days. No more blank checks. Now, it's a money order and the numbers are already filled in. They came up with a fancy name for this one too: prospective payment or fixed price per ailment, something they called DRGs or diagnostic related groups. Some patients thought DRG meant Discharge rapidly, gang. The picnic was over. From my point of view, the commodes had returned in full force.

We had gone from "We'll pay for whatever you get for whatever ails you no matter how many times you get it" to "We'll pay only so much for each kind of thing you get whenever you get it." The problem was people got it more often. Typically, they beat the system. Unit price increases leveled off some, but use rates went up. And so the policy works came up with yet another way to keep the growth of healthcare costs at manageable levels: "We'll pay only so much per year per person no matter what ails them, no matter what treatment they receive,

228

and no matter how often they receive it." Reformers called this reimbursement method capitation. Some hospital executives called it *decapitation.*

What unit discounts for volume purchases are to most businesses in the U.S. is what managed competition is to healthcare. Our alliance corporate staff is starkly aware of some of the unprecedented implications:

- Whereas before, hospitals may have lost dissatisfied patients over an extended period of time now they can lose a large group of patients overnight.
- Whereas before, and up to this day on the outpatient side of its business, hospitals received more revenues, the more units of services they actually provided to an individual patient; now they will be better off financially, given their fixed capitated payments, the fewer units of service they provide to individual patients.
- Whereas before, hospitals were induced by financial incentives to make people well, now the financial incentives are to keep people well.

CQI IN THE 1990s AND BEYOND: Some Final Thoughts

There are, of course, many other CQI implications from the radical changes that will result from managed competition. Hospital leaders serious about continuing to do a good job in a radically changed business will have to sort through them all and develop quality initiatives for the new business they will be bequeathed. There are several implications for our alliance's future quality efforts:

We will have to constantly remind ourselves that we now need to focus on continuous value improvement.

Many efforts to reduce costs do not improve quality. But many efforts to improve quality, do reduce costs. It is on these quality efforts that we need to concentrate our efforts. Quality and cost reduction are not anti-thetical ideas. When done with attention, quality endeavors can often reduce costs and prices. When we say CQI, we need to at least be thinking CVI (continuous value improvement). The American public is asking for more for less. We either need to tell them that it can't be done or mine the depths of our ingenuity to discover how it can be done.

Most of the alliance's employed physicians are family practice physicians.

The prime movers in this era crying out for prevention and for early detection are our primary care physicians. Sixty-five percent of our physicians are specialists. Thirty-five percent are family practice physicians. The direction of virtually all of health reform legislation is toward reversing these ratios. We work hard at maintaining healthy collaborative and mutually supportive relations with both of these kinds of physician groups during this period of radical change. The alignment of hospitals and family practice physicians will be relatively easy and natural because their collaboration will be in their transparent mutual self-interest. At the same time, we in the alliance will continue to extend ourselves as well to the specialists whose professional life is more rife with insecurity.

No institution is an island.

In the past, quality could often be delivered institution by institution. Value cannot be. Unity must emerge where duplication, waste, and inefficiency were structurally imbedded by separateness. It is no longer in anyone's self-interest to be alone. For perceptive leaders, the move will be from institutional quality to network value and strategic alliances. Old competitors will unite to face new competitors, often old collaborators. That's what the free market system we all celebrate is all about. In the future, you will be seeing many institutions going the route of the Susquehanna Healthcare System.

CQI requires a unity that encourages diversity, not a unity that requires uniformity.

In a previous chapter, I emphasized the need for continuity in continuous quality improvement. That idea is an easy one to lose sight of in a merger. The temptation is to impose successful elements of CQI on one's new partners.

At Muncy Valley Hospital, Divine Providence Hospital, and The Williamsport Hospital & Medical Center, employees share a rock-bed belief that we live and breathe for our patients and that our employees should be treated the way we ask them to treat our patients. At each hospital, institutional practices support this belief. Often, these practices have their own distinctive and attractive flavor—that deft special character that gives each hospital's expression of caring the feel of an invaluable and irreplaceable touch that can vivify a quality effort.

Muncy Valley Hospital is a down-to-earth, what-you-see-is-what-you-get, transparently honest homegrown hospital. It's a rural hospital in which every caregiver knows every patient and family member—often back a generation or two. Divine Providence provides a compassionate ambience infused by the spirit of those living out the implications of stewardship contained in the scriptures. At The Williamsport Hospital & Medical Center, employees faithfully practice the value of C.A.R.E. (courtesy, attentiveness, responsiveness, and empathy.)

Each hospital has a program with differing features to honor employees who habitually model the institution's value: at Muncy Valley and Divine Providence an employee of the month program; at The Williamsport Hospital & Medical Center, the C.A.R.E. employee of the month program. Each hospital also has a program to recognize individual acts of caring: at Muncy Valley, the take-five program; at Divine Providence the divine difference; at The Williamsport Hospital & Medical Center, the magic moment program. Instead of imposing any updated version of these programs on all institutions, we will continue these different expressions in their current form until that time when a grass-roots alliance expression emerges naturally.

As hospital consolidations, mergers and the creation of healthcare networks become the rule rather than the exception, satisfying the captive patient will be a new key indicator of successful CQI.

Each of our hospitals has a loyal clientele, some of whom are, to put it bluntly, partisan die-hards. One such person told me recently that she was anxious to find out "which disease was going where after the consolidation so that I can get the right disease when I get sick." Making her an enthusiastic customer when she gets the wrong disease will be the challenge. At the alliance, we already plan to include captive patient training in all our near-term programs.

Conclusion

Joel Barker, America's paradigm guru writes and speaks about paradigm shifters, paradigm pioneers, and paradigm settlers. Paradigm shifters are people who change the way business is done because it has become obsolete or irrelevant. Paradigm pioneers drive new paradigms from rough concept into practical application. Pioneer settlers try to play it safe in the old paradigm but land up being left behind by the paradigm pioneers.

We don't have to create America's healthcare paradigm. It's being, for better or for worse, created for us. Our challenge, once the new paradigm is established is to decide whether we are going to be paradigm pioneers or paradigm settlers. The fate of the paradigm settler is to be safe, secure, and over the long term, a failure. The most we can say to the settler is what a doctor once told a man in his fifties after a physical: "There's no reason why you can't live a completely normal life as long as you don't enjoy it." The destiny of the paradigm pioneer is fraught with risk and with promise. In healthcare, those who settle on past quality successes and on current quality models will watch things happen for a time, will likely get bored, and then wonder what happened. Paradigm pioneers . . . well they will enjoy—or struggle through—the experience of living out the ancient Chinese curse: "May you live in interesting times." One sure thing, paradigm pioneers will not be bored.

Throughout this book, I have contended that:

- **Success**—for the organization and for employees as professionals and persons *depends on*
- **Go-beyond quality**—that is customer-focused and directly related to their highest priority needs *ensured by*
- **A leadership team**—of corporate staff, department heads, and supervisors who are team builders, service managers, and servants *through*

- **A united workforce**—motivated, enabled, and empowered as individuals and as groups to *do their best by the customer in the*
- **Three dimensions of quality**—personal service, system convenience, and problem solution *because of a pervasively shared belief in*
- **Continuous value improvement**—that emphasizes high quality and competitive prices *so that*
- **Customers are well and happy**—what we in the final analysis hope will be the result of our serving the healthcare needs of the people in our community.

But, as Tom Peters says, "success invariably leads to hardening of the arteries." Things wear out. We believe that the prescription The Williamsport Hospital & Medical Center has followed during the past 10 years can help hospitals avoid the seemingly inevitable: organizational catheterization and the threat of institutional death.

A now defunct but once powerful airline had this slogan: "We earn our wings every day." Eastern's President, Frank Borman used to say: "Capitalism without bankruptcy is like Christianity without Hell." Well, several years ago, Eastern got its wings clipped and the airline went out of business. We at The Williamsport Hospital & Medical Center soberly acknowledge that not much in this world is built to last.

Yet in the chaos of the healthcare world today are opportunities for institutional renewal. Fortunately, we have been blessed with such an opportunity. Now that The Williamsport Hospital & Medical Center has joined Muncy Valley Hospital and Divine Providence Hospital in a new partnership called the Susquehanna Health System, we envision ourselves not at the end but at the beginning of our quality journey.

Appendix—Resources

Resource 2-A

"Remember the Shoe": Always Stay Focused on the Customer

We drive this thought home visually by using a shoe as a prop in the training and by having posters with the shoe and "Remember the Shoe" distributed in employee areas throughout the hospital in the first two years after these opening sessions.

A research corporation once asked several thousand people, "What are the most serious faults of people in business toward their customers?" In the same survey, they also asked, "What are the most serious faults of managers toward their employees?" The most common fault perceived by customers and employees turned out to be the same thing: *failure to see the other person's point of view.*

One of the reminders you'll hear often at TWH&MC is "Remember the Shoe." Know what it's like to walk in someone else's shoe. Be empathetic—that is, understand and appreciate the experience and perceptions of our customers and fellow employees.

"Remember Your Own Cookie Bag": Make Sure You C.A.R.E.

There once was a woman who was traveling from New York to London. She had been rushed all morning and hadn't eaten. When she got to JFK Airport, she noticed a fancy French bakery. She went in and bought a full bag of delicate cookies, took them with her luggage and sat down to wait for her plane.

She pulled a magazine out of her suitcase and, as she read, she reached over on the table and grabbed a cookie out of the bag and started to eat it. She noticed over the top of her magazine that there was a man across from her. He reached over the table and took a cookie. She couldn't believe it. So she took another cookie—and he took another cookie—she took another. Cookie after cookie they went through the bag until there was only one cookie left. Much to her amazement, he took the last cookie, broke it in half and gave half to her. He took the other half, smiled and walked away munching.

She did everything she could to restrain herself from blasting him right out of the airport. Then she heard the page for all passengers on

Flight 711 for London to bring their luggage to the check-in point. As the check-in clerk was moving her baggage through the scanner, there before her eyes was a completely filled bag of delicate French gourmet cookies.

The whole time she thought he was eating her cookies, she was eating his cookies!

As we often say here at TWH&MC, "Remember your own cookie bag!" If each of us C.A.R.E.s, all of us will C.A.R.E.; and when all of us C.A.R.E., we will be a great hospital. For a truly great hospital is one in which extremely small things are done extraordinarily well by virtually everybody almost all of the time.

"Remember Heaven & Hell": Practice 'Go-Beyond Quality' Service

A French author once described Heaven and Hell in a way that brings home the deepest meaning of C.A.R.E. Program. He described Hell as the most exquisite and inviting dining room imaginable. But when new residents of Hell sat down to eat, they made a shocking discovery: their elbows did not bend. And so they spent eternity the way they spent their time on earth: futilely trying to stuff themselves.

An adjoining banquet hall, which was Heaven, was just like Hell in every respect. And when new residents of Heaven sat down to eat, they also found out that their elbows did not bend. But, unlike the people in Hell, the people in Heaven spent eternity the way they spent their lives on earth: feeding the person across from them. Heaven or Hell?

A hospital, like almost any other place, can be like either Heaven or Hell for our patients and guests. It all depends on the degree to which we are willing to serve the needs of others, to bend over backwards and to do those little extra things that make our customers not just satisfied, but enthusiastic about us. Quality service is not just important . . . it is essential.

"Remember the Refrigerator": Quality Is a Together Thing

Two workmen were struggling unsuccessfully with a refrigerator at the threshold of a door. Finally after a half-hour of grunting and groaning, the fellow on the outside yelled to the fellow on the inside: "We're never going to get this damn refrigerator in." "In?" responded the fellow on the inside, "I've been trying to push it out."

As Casey Stengel once put it: "Getting good players signed up is easy. Getting them to play together—that's the hard part." It's the hard part of service excellence too.

Promise to C.A.R.E.

The C and the E of C.A.R.E. are the how of quality (Courtesy and Empathy). The A and the R are the what of quality, (Attentiveness and Responsiveness). All of the C.A.R.E. behaviors derive from these basic dispositions:

Courtesy means acting in a polite and considerate manner; explaining procedures, rules, and schedules to patients and fellow staff. What is routine for you is often quite mysterious and even frightening to others.

- Treat everyone as a special someone.
- Treat those who work with you or for you the way we ask you to treat guests.
- Show eagerness, interest, and pride in what you do. Be enthusiastic.
- Call adults Mr., Mrs., Miss, and their last name unless they let you know they'd prefer to be addressed otherwise.
- Make a good first impression. You never get a second chance to make a good first impression.
- Do everything you can to make all our guests feel comfortable— physically, mentally, and emotionally.
- Help make The Williamsport Hospital & Medical Center a pleasant place to work.

Our hospital is only as good as its people and the way we treat our patients. Around this hospital you'll find people of high ability and integrity. Superior people who care. People with trust and respect for the dignity of the individual. You're one of those people, too. That had a lot to do with your being hired. Be proud of what we are: A caring hospital.

*A*ttentiveness is really listening and hearing and being sensitive to other people's concerns and problems, their expressions of what they need and want. It's reading between the lines. Take time with people, listen to them, show your concern, make them feel special. They are, you know.

*R*esponsivenes is doing whatever and as much as you can to help another with a problem. Solve the problem if you can; get someone else to address the problem if you can't, follow up on all concerns. Don't leave anyone dangling.

*E*mpathy is showing others that you truly understand what they are saying and how they are feeling, learn how to paraphrase and reflect feelings, identify with others and their circumstances, let them know you really care. Showing that we care—that's the big challenge. It involves going out of our way to do little things and doing them *consistently*—little things like the following:

- Smiling and saying hello to patients, visitors, and fellow workers whenever you see them.
- Projecting a friendly nonverbal image to others.
- Practicing the 25 C.A.R.E. behaviors.

Note: We used an updated and adapted version of "C.A.R.E." Training developed by Personal and Professional Development, Inc., Chicago, Illinois, as a major source of much of the content for our kick off training.

Resource 2-B

Senior Management/Department Head Checklist

1. *Provides direction:*
   - Involves people in goal setting.
   - Establishes clear, challenging, and realistic goals.
   - Communicates these goals effectively.
   - Delegates responsibility and commensurate authority to the right people in the right way.
2. *Encourages open two-way communication:*
   - Regularly provides information needed to do job well.
   - Listens and learns from bad news.
   - Treats negative feedback as a gift.
   - Separates negative feedback from reaction.
   - Communicates up and down, honestly and positively.
   - Manages down as well as up.
3. *Coaches, supports his or her people, and facilitates their work:*
   - Measures own success by success of his or her team.
   - Teaches and develops new skills in team members.
   - Encourages, implements, and gives credit for ideas.
   - Provides people with:
     —Prioritized work.
     —Systems, procedures.
     —Resources to do their job well.
   - Backs them up.
4. *Gives objective feedback:*
   - Recognizes good performance more often than criticizes poor performance.
   - Relates rewards to performance.
   - Gives timely, specific feedback.
   - Overlooks the inconsequential.
   - Gives effective one-minute praise and one-minute reprimands.
   - "Good mouths" people.
5. *Follows up and follows through:*
   - Gets back to people.
   - Does not let important things fall in the cracks.

- Sees things through to successful conclusion.
- Attends to big payoff items.

6. *Hires the best people:*
   - Creates an environment that attracts people.
   - Knows how to define required skills.
   - Knows how to screen.
   - Knows how to interview.
   - Uses others in making selections.
   - Does not play favorites.

7. *Keeps bottom line in mind when making decisions:*
   - His or her team takes care of *customers* (task needs).
   - Treats quality as a part of productivity.
   - Personally takes care of *team,* including group maintenance and individual needs so the market will take care of you.
   - Integrates efforts with other departments.
   - Makes team feel part of the hospital's "Olympic team."

8. *Encourages innovation that works:*
   - Leads by liberating talent.
   - Creates climate that makes heroes of experimenters and "skunkwork."
   - Encourages calculated risks.

9. *Gives subordinates clear-cut decisions when they're needed:*
   - Practices try it, fix it, do it, drop it methods.
   - Tolerates—sometimes even rewards—failure.
   - Is purposely impatient with inaction.

10. *Shows a high level of integrity:*
    - Treats employees the way we want them to treat customers.
    - Has the respect of superior and subordinates alike.
    - Tries to mesh personal and organizational needs and goals.

11. *Is committed to excellence:*
    - Fosters excitement and pride in team.
    - Manages self well.
    - Promotes, models, and teaches self-management.

12. *Sees leadership role as service not team members as subservient:*
    - Views his or her role as helping others get their work done—not the other way around (MBWA).
    - Sees people as the job; paper as an interruption.

Resource 2-C
CQI Manual's Table of Contents

Resource 2-D.
Sample Departmental Service Plan

DEPARTMENT: ANESTHESIA   SERVICE STRATEGIES: You'll have our undivided attention.

KEY CUSTOMER SERVICES PROVIDED:

General anesthesia, monitored anesthesia care, informed consent, reassure patient.

CUSTOMER	MOMENT OF TRUTH	CUSTOMER EXPECTATIONS/NEEDS	SERVICE PLAN (Who, What, When, Where, How)
Patients	M_1 Pre-op visit	Explain what type of anesthesia they will receive, what will be done, and when.	Who—M.D. or C.R.N.A. What—Pre-op visit. When—1. When patient comes in for PAT. 2. Day prior to surgery for in-house patients. 3. Morning of surgery for early AM admissions. Where—1. Patient room. 2. Conference room 2-A How—1. Identify self and position. 2. Identify patient. 3. Obtain history. a. Complete Pre-assessment sheet with available information. 4. Obtain informed consent. a. Explain type of anesthesia patient will receive. b. Explain risks. c. Explain monitoring equipment to help allay fears. 5. Explain what will happen upon arrival in OR. a. Identification. b. IV

247

CUSTOMER	MOMENT OF TRUTH	CUSTOMER EXPECTATIONS/NEEDS	SERVICE PLAN (Who, What, When, Where, How)
Patients	M₂ Arrival in OR	A. Needs to be reassured. B. Needs to know what will be done to them.	Who—C.R.N.A. or M.D. What—Pre-anesthetic care When—Upon arrival Where—Holding area How—1. Identify patient, greet by name. 2. Verify surgeon and surgery. 3. Complete any forms as required. 4. Explain what will be done. 5. Start IV. 6. Answer any questions. 7. Estimate waiting time
	M₃ Anesthesia induction		Who—C.R.N.A. or M.D. What—Induce anesthesia When—Upon arrival of surgeon Where—Scheduled operating room How—1. Transport patient to OR. 2. Identify patient in OR. 3. Move to bed unless induction is done on OR litter. 4. Attach all monitoring equipment. a. Explain each item to patient. 5. Give appropriate anesthesia agents. 6. Maintain appropriate anesthesia level throughout surgery
	M₄ Post-op		Who—C.R.N.A. or M.D. What—Post-op care When—Anesthesia is finished

CUSTOMER	MOMENT OF TRUTH	CUSTOMER EXPECTATIONS/NEEDS	SERVICE PLAN (Who, What, When, Where, How)
Patients	M₄ Post-op		*Where*—OR—Recovery room patient care area. *How*—1. Transfer patient to recovery room. a. If not open, patient is recovered by anesthetist. 2. Give completed report to recovery room nurse. a. If not open, give report to R.N. on patient care area after recovery of patient by anesthetist. 3. Post-op visit (within 24 hours of anesthesia). a. Greet patient by name. b. Introduce yourself. c. Discuss patient's condition. d. Ask if there is anything you can do for them. e. Write Post-op note to contain. (1) Date. (2) Time. (3) Post-op condition. (4) Signature

Resource 3-A.
Appreciation Review Guidelines

THE WILLIAMSPORT HOSPITAL & MEDICAL CENTER

EXPERIMENTAL
APPRECIATION/MERIT PAY
REVIEW FOR SUPERVISORS

EMPLOYEE NAME _____

EMPLOYEE NUMBER _____

DEPARTMENT _____

TITLE _____

POSITION CODE NUMBER _____

COST CENTER NUMBER _____

DATE _____
(ANNIVERSARY DATE MO/DAY/CURRENT YEAR)

GENERAL DIRECTIONS

I. **Agreeing on Expectations—Performance Plan**

The purpose of an appreciation review is to improve employee performance. Employees need to know exactly what areas of responsibility they will be reviewed on during the evaluation period ending June 30 of each fiscal year.

Please meet with each employee before the beginning of the evaluation period to develop a specific agreed upon set of expectations in these three key areas:

A. The employee's job description.

B. Special assignments or projects (workplans—living job descriptions may be used for these special projects).

C. Relational responsibility (the C.A.R.E. behaviors may be used here).

The end result of this meeting is a common understanding of exact job expectations for this evaluation period. Therefore, assign priorities and give the employee a written set of expectations.

On-Going Verbal Feedback

During the review period, you should reinforce good efforts and encourage improvements through day-to-day contact with employees. Changing conditions may result in changes in the activities performed by the employee. Record these on this form. Also be sure to record specific incidents that describe performance and place in the employee's working file.

**REGULAR VERBAL FEEDBACK
IS THE MOST IMPORTANT PART
OF THIS PROCESS.**

II. Appreciation review

This formal meeting should be:

A. A summary

B. Positive when possible, constructively critical when necessary

C. A two-way exchange of information

D. Future oriented

Therefore, the time allotted should approximate these guidelines: <u>R.A.P.</u>

R — Review the past (25%)

A — Assess the present (15%)

P — Plan the future (60%)

The attached suggested agenda will help assure that you follow these guidelines. Key areas for the evaluation period should be assigned. Initial ratings and comments may be made by the employee, or by the supervisor before the session. Final ratings should be arrived at through discussion. Mock merit raises will be calculated by multiplying the summary rating by the maximum allowable increase.

PERS-2753-A

I. PERFORMANCE PLAN

A. JOB DESCRIPTION (Main Duties and Responsibilities)
Attach Page 1 of Position Description

PERS-2753-A Rev. 11/87

254

B. SPECIAL PROJECTS:

PERS-2753-A Rev. 11/87

255

C. INTERPERSONAL/MANAGERIAL RELATIONS: Courtesy, Attentiveness, Responsiveness, Enthusiasm (Complete the list of C.A.R.E behaviors on page 15 if applicable)
Summarize, rate and comment on these aspects of C.A.R.E behaviors below:

1. Relationships with Patients and Guests

2. Relationships with others in the Department

a. Fellow-employees

b. Supervisor(s)

PERS-2753-A Rev. 11/87

3. Relationships with Employees in other Departments

4. Relationships with Physicians

II. AREAS FOR IMPROVEMENT	PLAN FOR IMPROVEMENT

PERS-2753-A Rev. 11/87

III. PERFORMANCE SUMMARY RATING

Indicate the overall performance rating which best reflects achievements described earlier and recommend merit increase.

		MERIT INCREASE RANGE
☐	Results achieved consistently met requirements of the job in all key areas of responsibility and exceeded them in some.	90-100%
☐	Results achieved met the requirements of the job in all key areas of responsibility.	75-89%
☐	Results achieved met the requirements of the job in some key areas but not in others.	50-74%
☐	Written Warning - Results achieved did not meet the requirements of the job in many areas of responsibility.	0

Recommended Merit Increase [   ]

IV. JUSTIFICATION FOR PERFORMANCE SUMMARY RATING

PERS-2753-A Rev. 11/87

259

V. EMPLOYEE COMMENTS

The employee's signature simply indicates that his/her performance was discussed with him/her. It is not an indication that there is agreement with the results.

Employee Signature: _____ Date: _____

Supervisor Signature: _____ Date: _____

Department Head Signature: _____ Date: _____

Corporate Signature: _____ Date: _____

PERS-2753-A Rev. 11/87

Resource 3-B.
Motivating Employees:
Applying the Principles

I. Content Models

A) Maslow's Hierarchy of Needs

1. People are wanting beings whose needs can influence their behavior.
2. A person's needs are arranged in an order of importance from basic needs like food and shelter to complex needs like self-esteem and achievement.
3. A person advances from one level of the hierarchy—from basic to complex needs—only when the lower need is minimally satisfied (satisfaction progression).
4. Satisfied needs do not act as motivators.
5. Only unsatisfied needs can influence behavior.
6. *Motivate by appealing to unsatisfied needs.*

B) Herzberg's Two-Factor Theory

1. There are two different kinds of factors in the relationship between a supervisor and subordinates.
2. The painkillers (or as Herzberg calls them the "hygiene factors") are aspects of the job environment and relate to lower-level needs in the Maslow hierarchy.
3. Painkillers are related to the way the job environment provides for the basic security and social needs of its employees (e.g., money, security, rest periods, benefits, friendly atmosphere, clean conditions). They reduce sources of dissatisfaction.
4. Painkillers do not motivate people to work any harder than is necessary to hold their job.
5. The Turn-ons or motivators are a set of conditions intrinsic to the job itself.

6. They draw out extra effort on the part of employees and tend to increase performance capacity.
7. The Turn-ons relate to higher-level needs like the need for achievement, recognition, challenge, responsibility, and growth.
8. The Turn-ons excite people and motivate them to tap their energies to contribute to greater organizational effectiveness.
9. *Use Turn-ons not Painkillers to motivate.*

C) Alderfer's ERG Theory

1. People have three categories of need: a) existence needs (E)—Maslow's basic and security needs; 2) relatedness (R)—Maslow's social or belonging needs; and 3) growth (G)—Maslow's achievement and self-actualization.
2. The less each level is satisfied, the more it will be desired.
3. The more lower-level needs are satisfied, the greater the desire for higher-level needs (satisfaction progression).
4. The less the higher-levels needs have been satisfied, the more the lower-level needs will be desired (need frustration).
5. More than one need may be operative at one time.
6. *Motivate at a) level of current need; b) progressive levels as lower levels are met; c) the next lower level when a higher level is frustrated; and d) all levels of currently felt needs.*

II. Process Models

A) Expectancy Theory

1. People behave in various ways because they expect to satisfy certain needs.
2. Expectations are usually a matter of probabilities.
3. Whether and how well a person performs a certain act depends on three factors:
   - Will what I want satisfy a need (instrumentality)?
   - How likely is it that I will obtain what I want by what I plan to do (confidence)?

- Is it worth the effort? How valuable is it to me to make an effort to satisfy this need when I have other needs and limited energy (valence)?
4. *Motivate by clarifying worker expectations and rewards and by adjusting them to each other.*

B) Equity Theory

1. Workers compare the differences between what they and other reference persons bring to or put into their work (e.g., effort, skills, education, task performance) and what they get out of their work (e.g., pay, promotion, recognition, status).
2. People are motivated to reduce their efforts when they think they are not being fairly rewarded for their work in comparison to others like them.
3. *Motivate through reward systems that are fair to the same kinds of employees at comparable performance levels.*

III.   Reinforcement Theory

Type of Reinforcement	Purpose	Result
Rewards for jobs well done (positive reinforcement)	Get people to keep up good work	Frequently effective when properly done
Threat of undesired consequences (negative reinforcement)	Get people to keep up good work	Best if applied progressively
Punishment	Get people to stop undesirable behavior	Unpredictable: may cause behavior to cease; may cause employee to avoid getting caught but not cease the undesirable behavior itself

Type of Reinforcement	Purpose	Result
Removal of rewards (extinction)	Get people to stop undesirable behavior	Not too applicable; does discourage previously encouraged behaviors.

1. Positive reinforcement (rewards for jobs well done):
   - Causes behavioral changes in desired directions.
   - Enhances the worker's self-image.
2. Negative reinforcement (punishment, threat of undesired consequences):
   - May produce strange, unpredictable, and undesirable behavior.
   - May motivate worker to avoid getting caught.
3. Employees react positively when rewards are contingent upon work behavior.
4. Employees react negatively when rewards are not contingent upon work behavior.
5. Decreased motivation and performance occur when employees are not rewarded as a matter of practice.
6. Guidelines for giving positive reinforcement:
   - Tie rewards to performance.
   - Give rewards as soon as possible after performance.
   - Don't reserve rewards to extraordinary accomplishments; give for smaller achievements too.
   - There are many rewards that don't cost money; use them.
   - Reward people intermittently and unpredictably rather than continuously and at fixed intervals (variable ratio schedule).
   - Don't underestimate the value of small rewards.

Resource 4-A.
Nuts & Bolts I

Based on *Service America* by Ron Zemke & Karl Albrecht and *Service Excellence* (tape) by Ron Zemke

Session 1: The Customer

1. Customers are the center of a service organization's existence. A critical measure of quality is customer satisfaction.
2. How you think the customer perceives you and how the customer perceives you can be a mile apart.
3. We must not only provide good service. We must work to make sure the customers perceive that they are getting good service.
4. Customers' needs and expectations change over time. Customer satisfaction begins and ends with understanding and acting on the customer's changing needs and expectations.
5. A key to staying close to the customer is naïve listening. Ask your customers what they need and want and are willing to pay for.
6. Customers are concerned about their immediate needs, not our operational difficulties.
7. Customers:
   - Are *need-driven*—we need to know their needs, expectations, attitudes, and wants.
   - Have *options*—they don't have to come here. They can go elsewhere.
   - Have *portable loyalties*—customer loyalty is fragile, circumstantial, fleeting. It is satisfied only by a continuously satisfying level of service.
8. The customer's perception of our hospital can be:
   - Measured.
   - Improved by managing the moments of truth in accordance with customer expectations.

Session 2: The Service Triangle

1. *Customer Satisfaction*—Customers develop mental report cards on a hospital with grades based on whether their needs are met during the moments of truth with the hospital's employees—on whether they perceive they have received quality service.
2. *Service Management*—Quality service doesn't just happen; it is consciously managed. The service management process must begin with a clear understanding of the wants and needs of the customer. Service begins and ends with the customer. The customer is the key to defining the services of a service-focused business. There are three elements to the service management process:
   - A well-conceived *service strategy* derives from the customer and from what he wants. The service strategy is the definition of what we want to do to, for, and with the customer. It is the vision of what we are trying to create for the customer through our hospital's services.
   - The *service systems* have to deliver what is in the service strategy and is a focused response to customer needs. The service delivery systems are the way we deploy the resources at our disposal to meet customer needs.
   - *Service people* must know how to use the service systems and must clearly see the role they play in the service strategy. There are two types of service people: those who work on the front line and meet and serve customers and those who serve those who serve customers.

Session 3: The Service Strategy

1. A service strategy is a touchstone or vision that describes and helps everyone remember and deliver on what our hospital and your service area are trying to do for the customer.
2. The basic approach to any service strategy is to hear any burden, pay any price to carry out the promise we make to the customer in the statement of our service strategy.

3. The essential elements of a service strategy are:
   - A non-trivial statement:
     —Not an empty advertising slogan.
     —Has ramifications within the organization.
     —Congruent with our marketing strategy.
   - That makes a noticeable difference:
     —Is clearly seen.
     —Understood as a difference.
   - Has value in the customer's eyes:
     —Really important to customer.
     —Speaking for himself.
4. The service strategy represents your company's approach to satisfying the customer.
5. Your service strategy should differentiate you from the competition.
6. The service strategy should be one that is deliverable by your service area and your organization.
7. The service strategy must not be an afterthought; it must *be* the thought.

Session 4: Service Systems

1. A service system is the integrated and purposeful organization, use, and management of all the resources (money, equipment, facilities, time) and methodical procedures that service people have at their disposal to exceed the needs of customers.
2. A service delivery system is an organization's approach to making good on its promise to the customer.
3. To be effective, it must:
   - Be designed to accommodate the user.
   - Meet the reasonable expectations of the provider.
   - Include a feedback loop to make it self-correcting.
4. Several things are necessary in designing an effective service delivery system:
   - Understanding the cycle of services.
   - Plotting the course of our customers' moments of truth.

- Organizing, orchestrating, and deploying our resources methodically to satisfy the customer's expressed desires for each moment of truth in each service cycle.

Session 5: Service People

1. People are the most visible part of service.
2. Quality service depends on empowering people to work on the customer's behalf.
3. It's easy to confuse a poor system with poor people performance. Good people can't deliver quality services with bad systems.
4. It is also easy to underestimate the amount of training and monitoring it takes to implement a customer-responsive service strategy.
5. People need to be carefully taught:
   - The moments of truth.
   - Customer expectations for these moments.
   - The meaning of service strategy.
   - The way to make the system work.
6. There are two kinds of people in a service business: those who serve the customer and those who serve those who serve the customer.
7. There are two kinds of people who serve the customer:
   - *Primary* service people—Their job descriptions explicitly describe their direct contact responsibilities for the customer (for example, nursing personnel and all other caregivers).
   - *Secondary* service people—In the course of their daily work, they come into contact with patients even though their explicit assignments do not emphasize customer relations (for example, maintenance mechanics and other support people).

Resource 4-B.
Nuts & Bolts II

Based on *At America's Service* by Karl Albrecht

1. The Service Revolution:
   - The United States revives its quality legacy.
   - The way to deliver great service.
   - The seven sins of service delivery.
2. Service Management:
   - What it is.
   - Key moments of truth and the service triangle.
   - World-class quality.
3. Off to a Flying Stop:
   - Quality as a marathon, not a sprint.
   - Staying the course.
   - Avoiding fads.
4. Common Mistakes:
   - Poor customer focus.
   - Unmotivated employees.
   - All foam, no beer.
5. Common Pitfalls:
   - Counterculture.
   - Poor work environment.
   - Senior, middle management's lack of leadership.
6. The Manufacturing Model Does Not Work:
   - Why.
   - Examples.
   - The new way to go.
7. Toward a New Service Model:
   - Changing the model.
   - The service culture.
   - Managers as servants; employees as bosses.
8. Internal Service:
   - Your internal customers.
   - Coordination, collaboration, consolidation.
   - Managing internal service.

9. Implementing Service Management:
   - Service versus cost.
   - Applying institutional resources.
   - The basics.
10. Phase I: Understand Your Customer.
   - Don't assume.
   - Customer perception.
   - Measure service.
11. Phase II: Clarify Your Service Strategy:
   - Repeat: What it is.
   - How to set it.
   - How not to set it.
12. Phase III: Educate Employees:
   - Wall-to-wall training.
   - Orientation.
   - Communication.
13. Phase IV: Implement Grass-Roots Improvements:
   - Department head leadership.
   - Improving systems.
   - Plant many seeds?—We say no.
14. Phase V: Make It Last:
   - Hire the best.
   - Give right incentives.
   - Measure and give feedback.
15. Preach the Gospel:
   - The starting point: the top.
   - Determination, patience.
   - Earn wings every day.

Resource 4-C.
Closing the Service Gaps

Session 1: Total Quality Management

1. Total quality management (TQM) is a scientific method of ensuring the delivery of legendary service by:
   - Setting up the service systems.
   - Teaching them to employees.
   - Monitoring the execution of service.
   - Relaying customer feedback.
   - Rewarding or constructively criticizing so that, superior technical service and exemplary personal service are delivered and experienced.
2. The old quality standard was:
   What customers expect equals what they receive.
3. The new quality standard is go-beyond or legendary quality:
   What customers get exceeds what they expect.
4. Customers expect two things of every service:
   - Their problem is solved.
   - They have a good experience.
5. There is simultaneity between the delivery of a service and the reception of a service that does not exist between the making and the use of a product. What are the service implications?
6. The five things people judge about a service are:
   - Reliability.
   - Tangibles.
   - Assurance.
   - Responsiveness.
   - Empathy.
7. The single most important measure of quality is the lasting subjective satisfaction of the customer.
8. Customers evaluate three dimensions of every hospital service:
   - The interpersonal dimension—how they are treated (C.A.R.E.).
   - The systems dimension—how hassle-free service is (TQM).

- The outcome dimension—the solution of their problem (MEDIMPROVE).
9. To exceed customers expectations in these three dimensions, we must manage:
   - Technical performance.
   - Relational behavior.
   - The reality of quality (actually delivered).
   - The perception of quality (subjectively appreciated).
10. We must therefore manage the quality of two relationships:
    - Managers and employees.
    - Employees and customers.

Session 2: Understanding Customer Expectations

1. Customers develop their service expectations from four sources:
   - Word of mouth.
   - Personal needs.
   - Past experience.
   - External communications of service business.
2. The most important service gap to be eliminated is the gap between customers' expectations and their perception of the service.
3. This gap—what we refer to as *the* gap—usually exists when the customer and the providers have different ideas about what's really important in a service.
4. Most needed—an ongoing process to determine the features in services considered important by the customer and the level of these features expected by customers.
5. Gap 1: The first of the gaps causing *the* gap is not really knowing what customers expect: Managers have a different perception of what customers expect than what customers actually expect.
6. Being just a little wrong about customer expectations could mean losing customers, spending money on things customers do not want, and even losing in a competitive environment.
7. The challenge is to close gap 1 by installing systems that ensure accurate, up-to-date information about customer expectations.

Session 3: The Right Service Quality Standards and Service Systems

1. Gap 2: A second gap causing *the* gap is the failure to accurately translate real customer expectations into the right service standards.
2. Maintaining service quality depends on:
   - Recognizing customers' desires.
   - Establishing the right standards.
   - Having people willing and able to meet the service standards.
3. Gap 3: The third gap causing *the* gap is the gap between service standards and service delivery systems caused by inappropriate, inadequate, or uncoordinated resources.
4. Develop the right service delivery systems by installing, managing, and orchestrating the needed resources.
5. Gap 4: The fourth gap causing *the* gap is communicating what is not being delivered.
6. Accurately reflect what the customer receives in the service encounter.
7. Some musts for the rest of the 90s:
   - Develop blueprints, detailed maps, or flow charts of processes and systems.
   - Identify fail points—that is, places in the process where deficiencies are likely to occur.
   - Design quality into the process when it can be done best—when it's first taking shape.
   - Combine high-tech with high touch.
   - Differentiate services.
   - Seek constant improvement.
   - Do the service right the first time.
   - Do the service very right the second time.
   - Measure.

Resource 5-A.
MEDIMPROVE CQI Project Guidelines for Developing Patient-Management Guidelines

I. Purpose and objectives
   A. Define the reasons for developing patient-management guidelines (PMG): reduce inappropriate care and improve patient outcomes.
   B. Define the desired outcomes of patient-management guidelines: achieve or surpass results of benchmark programs.
   C. Delineate the methods for implementing patient-management guidelines.
   D. Identify and rank the diseases for which patient-management guidelines are to be developed in accordance with JCAHO standards (i.e., for high-volume, high-cost, problem-prone concerns) and the hospital's strategic goals and patient service priorities.
   E. Over time develop comprehensive patient-management guidelines:
      1. Prehospital.
      2. Emergency department.
      3. Inpatient days from day 1 to the end of the stay:
         • Medical/surgical floors.
         • Special units (e.g. ICU, CCU, IMC).
         • Admission criteria to special units.
      4. Discharge planning.
   F. Focus on optimal clinical outcomes, not on maximizing revenues or minimizing lengths of stay.
   G. Emphasize on key activities, interventions, testing, and therapies that are critical to patient outcomes, not everything that can be done for the patient.

    H. Include a mechanism for monitoring and documenting variance from guidelines and reasons for variance with any corrective actions necessary.

    I. Sequence activities so that important tasks (for example, physical therapy and occupational therapy) are completed simultaneously when possible and in the proper order to optimize length of stay.

II. Focus and format

    A. Select a process that is measurable and narrow enough in scope so as to be susceptible to improvement.

    B. Develop a standardized format for patient-management guidelines throughout the institution.

    C. Make sure all patient-management guidelines follow the standard format.

III. Benchmarks and reference materials

    A. Use internal and external benchmarks to develop the beginning frameworks for patient-management guidelines.

    B. Obtain reference material to support improvement of the selected processes:

        1. Other hospital departments.

        2. Neighboring hospitals.

        3. Literature on clinical pathways, algorithms, practice parameters, practice and treatment protocols.

        4. American Medical Association, American Hospital Association, The Voluntary Hospitals of America.

IV. Composition of PMG team

    A. Include members from all the disciplines involved in the selected patient's care.

    B. Involve medical, clinical, and management representatives on all teams. Select a physician as an advocate and process proponent with other members of the medical staff.

    C. Manage the barriers to physician involvement:

        1. Physician time constraints.

        2. Management's indifference to physician perspective.

        3. Differences in terminology and for problem-solving approaches.

    D. Include a facilitator in CQI tools and team dynamics to maintain focus and resolve conflicts.

  E. Involve patients in the process for developing guidelines by using patient satisfaction surveys, focus groups, and direct interviews.

  F. Ensure administrative support with data collection and analysis and clerical personnel.

  G. Empower team members to directly communicate with any appropriate information source including customers, suppliers, executive leadership, and support personnel.

  H. Develop flow diagrams for the service process being developed and ensure complete team understanding.

V. Developing patient-management guidelines

  A. Start by flowcharting the current process and flagging areas of high variability.

  B. Foster decisions that are consensus (win-win) oriented and focus on delivering value (i.e., improvements in quality and reduction in costs) to the process.

  C. Establish realistic timetables for accomplishment of team activities, including adequate meeting schedules and deadlines for reporting ongoing progress and final results.

  D. Consult any needed experts before finalization.

VI. Implementation and evaluation

  A. Present the patient-management guidelines to involved medical staff and nursing departments, the executive committee of the medical staff, the medical staff, as well as the MEDIMPROVE committee and the patient care committee of the hospital's board of managers.

  B. Use information to educate not punish or sanction.

  C. Implement the patient-management guidelines on a pilot basis (e.g., on one or two selected floors or units) before general implementation.

  D. Apply the mechanisms for monitoring and documenting variance from the guidelines.

  E. Identify the reasons for the variance and corrective actions.

  F. Whenever possible, make the patient-management guidelines part of the patient charting system.

  G. Recognize and reward organizational, team, and individual successes.

Resource 5-B. Sample Patient-Management Guideline: Total Knee Arthroscopy

	DAY 1	DAY 2	DAY 3
PHYSICIAN: (M.D.)			
ASSESSMENT	Treatment Plan H & P Nutrition/diet	Medical stability	
INTERVENTION	CPM Ice PRN Routine ortho. orders Set staple removal	A.M. rounds	A.M. rounds
	(date) diet as per T&R		
NURSING (N):			
ASSESSMENT	Medical history Baseline physical condition PROM Elimination Pain	Bathing needs Comfort/pain Skin/wound q. shift, PROM Elimination	FIMS—adm.
INTERVENTION	Complete data base Set pain med sched. CPM bid—chart Est. date of last BM	Review comfort measures Review Knee align. Tub/shower/ sponge bath— issue equip. CPM qid, increase 10° daily—chart Ice PRN Pain med schedule in place BM w/in last 48 hrs.	Complete FIMS adm assessment

	DAY 1	DAY 2	DAY 3
O.T.: ASSESSMENT	Transfers	Transfers ADLs Driving W/C mobility	Homemaking Adm. FIMS ADLs
INTERVENTION	Transfer bed/ chair/toilet	Complete init. eval. Initiate ADL program Pt. referred to ortho surg re: driving Transfers tub/ shower instruct nursing, Instruct pt. in W/C use A.M. ADLs	Set homemaking program w/pt. Complete adm. FIMS assess. A.M. ADLs
P.T.: ASSESSMENT	Ambulation/WBS ROM W/C fit Amb. transfers	ROM LE ex. limitations Ambulation	Ambulation FIMS adm. Pain control
INTERVENTION	Amb. room distance, ROM (act. & pass.)—set baseline Provide approp. W/C Sit/stand transfers w/AWD.	Set up LE ex. program Send walking device to all areas Init. assess. complete	ROM & LE ex. program Amb. levels/non- levels Complete adm. FIMS
T.R.: ASSESSMENT INTERVENTION		Initial assess. Leisure skills assess.	Adm. FIMS Complete adm. FIMS

	DAY 1	DAY 2	DAY 3
PSYCHOLOGY: ASSESSMENT INTERVENTION			
SOC. SVCS.: ASSESSMENT INTERVENTION	Initiate assess.	D/C plan	D/C plan Establish D/C plan Complete assess.
D/C PLANNING & PATIENT EDU.	Pt. oriented to clinical path. (ALL) Pt. view "Orient. to Rehab" video (N) Review avail. comfort measures (N) Review WBS w/pt. (PT) Review proper transfer tech. (OT)	Review comfort measures (N) Review knee align. (N) Review ADL equip. needs w/patient (OT)	Review strategies for post D/C leisure/ community activity (TR)
TESTS/ PROCEDURES	Protime, if not already drawn	Protimes	Protimes
MEDS	Anticoagulant Analgesic Meds per T&R/ report	Anticoagulant Analgesic	Anticoagulant Analgesic
CONSULTS	PT/OT/TR/SS		

281

	DAY 1	DAY 2	DAY 3
KEY PATIENT OUTCOMES	Pt. demonstrates: • amb.—min. assist w/AWD & maintain WBS (PT) • Transfer w/ min. assist, maintain WBS (OT) • tolerance of ROM program (PT) • verbal understanding of rehab routine (N) • verbal understanding of pain control (N)	Pt. demonstrates: • bathing— min. assist w/adaptive equip. (N) • adeq. pain control (N) • tolerance of TKA ex. & ROM program (PT) • safe, indep. use of W/C for functional use on 3 West (OT)	Pt. demonstrates: • amb. levels 150' w/supv./ AWD (PT) • amb. non-levels mod. assist/AWD (PT) • tolerance to TKA ex. & ROM program with sched. meds and comfort measures (PT) • min. assist w/home-making tasks (OT) • verbal confirmation tentative D/C plan (S/S)
PHYSICIAN: ASSESSMENT INTERVENTION	Post D/C therapy Meds for D/C Write meds for D/C Write post D/C therapy prescription	D/C patient D/C Summary Copy D/C summ. to ref./family M.D.	
NURSING: ASSESSMENT INTERVENTION	Meds D/C FIMS Write meds for D/C Complete D/C FIMS	Equip. for D/C Post D/C appointments	

	DAY 1	DAY 2	DAY 3
O.T.: ASSESSMENT INTERVENTION	D/C FIMS Complete D/C FIMS D/C from O.T.		
P.T.: ASSESSMENT	D/C FIMS LE & ROM ex. program	ROM	
INTERVENTION	Complete D/C FIMS Review LE & ROM home ex. program		
T.R.: ASSESSMENT INTERVENTION	D/C FIMS Complete D/C FIMS D/C T.R.		
PSYCHOLOGY: ASSESSMENT INTERVENTION			
SOC. SVCS.: ASSESSMENT	Post D/C community services		
INTERVENTION	Review D/C plans w/pt.		

	DAY 1	DAY 2	DAY 3
D/C PLANNING & PATIENT EDU.	Review med. ed. w/pt. (N) Schedule ortho. appt. (N) Pt. given written home LE & ROM ex. program (PT) Initiate post D/C referrals (ALL)	Pt. given written follow-up appts. (N)	
TESTS/ PROCEDURES	Protimes		
MEDS	Anticoagulant Analgesic	D/C anticoagulant Analgesic	
CONSULTS			
KEY PATIENT OUTCOMES	Patient demonstrates: • verbal understanding of D/C meds (N) • verbal understanding of D/C plans (S/S) • adequate leisure life skills (TR) • verbal understanding of leisure activities for continued therapeutic gains (TR)	Patient demonstrates: • AROM (10°–90°) PROM) (5°–100°) (PT) • discharged on time (N) • discharged w/all equip./ prescriptions/ & written follow-up appts. (N)	

	DAY 1	DAY 2	DAY 3
PHYSICIAN: ASSESSMENT INTERVENTION	Comfort Eval. pt.'s tolerance to TKA LE ex. ROM program AM Rounds	AM Rounds	AM Rounds
NURSING: ASSESSMENT INTERVENTION	Comfort Skin/wound ROM		PROM Bathing Skin/wound Ortho. complication
O.T.: ASSESSMENT INTERVENTION	Home eval. /home TX Discuss home eval./Tx need w/PT	Homemaking ADLs Transfers D/C ADL program	Equip. needs Tub transfers Review tub transfers w/pt.— issue handout
P.T.: ASSESSMENT INTERVENTION	ROM Home eval/home TX LE & ROM ex. program Car transfer Discuss home eval./Tx need w/OT Establish home ex. program	ROM Ambulation— levels/non- levels LE & ROM ex. program Non-levels (ramps/curbs/ steps) Review LE & home ex. program w/pt.	Equip. needs Post D/C therapy need Ambulation non-levels Discuss post D/C Tx w/pt. (VNA/ outpt.)

	DAY 1	DAY 2	DAY 3
T.R.: ASSESSMENT INTERVENTION		Commun. transition Commun. reintegration	
PSYCHOLOGY: ASSESSMENT INTERVENTION			
SOC. SVCS.: ASSESSMENT INTERVENTION		D/C plan Need for care giver inst. Review staff conf. w/pt./care giver	Post D/C follow-up needs w/pt. Coord. D/C follow up w/PT and pt. (VNA/outpt.)
D/C PLANNING & PATIENT EDU.	Review D/C instr. pamphlet— wound care & ortho complications (N) Review ROM & home ex. program w/pt. (PT)	Staff conference (ALL) Review equip. needs w/pt. (ALL)	Finalize & arrange for all equip. needs (ALL)
TESTS/ PROCEDURES	Protimes	Protimes	Protimes
MEDS	Anticoagulant Analgesic	Anticoagulant Analgesic	Anticoagulant Analgesic
CONSULTS			

	DAY 1	DAY 2	DAY 3
KEY PATIENT OUTCOMES	Patient demonstrates: • skin/wound free of redness & drainage (N) • indep. in proper knee align (N) • indep. in comfort measures (N) • CPM 80° (N) • AROM 10°–75° (PT) • CPM 80° (N) • AROM 10°–75° (PT) • PROM 10°–80° (PT) • verbal understanding of ROM & home ex. program (PT) • car transfer w/supv. (PT)	Patient demonstrates: • indep. in home-making needs (OT) • indep. in ADL program (OT) • amb. levels indep. 150' w/AWD; non-levels min. assist (PT) • Transfer indep. W/C/ toilet/bed (OT) • indep. w/ home ex. program (PT) • confidence in accessing community resources (TR)	Patient demonstrates: • CPM 110° (N) • bathing indep. (N) • indep. in skin/ wound care (N) • verbal understanding of ortho complications (N) • verbal understanding of equip. needs & acquisition (ALL) • amb. non-levels w/supv. & AWD (PT) • D/C plans finalized (S/S) • tub transfer w/min. assist & AWD (OT)

Resource 6-A

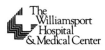

The Williamsport Hospital & Medical Center

C.A.R.E. EMPLOYEE NOMINATION

FROM: _____   _____
            (Nominator/Nominators)   (Date)

_____   _____
            (Department)   (Job Title)

TO: _____
            (Dept. Head)

SUBJECT: C.A.R.E. Employee of the Month Nomination

I have read the C.A.R.E. Criteria and respectfully nominate

_____
        (Name)   (Job Title)   (Division)

for consideration as the C.A.R.E. Employee of the Month. The reasons for this nomination are:

_____
_____
_____
_____
_____
_____
_____
_____
_____
_____
_____
_____
_____
_____
_____
_____

(PLEASE COMPLETE IN BLACK INK)   PERS-2759 Rev. 10/92

289

_____

INSTRUCTIONS

1. Supervisor submit nomination to Department Head within five days after end of month.
2. Department Head submit approved nominations to Administrative Representatives within three days after receipt from Supervisor.
3. Administrative Representative submit approved nominations to C.A.R.E. Committee, c/o Human Resources Department, within two days after receipt from the Department Head.

Department Head Comments:

_____

_____

_____

_____

_____

_____

☐ Nomination Approved   Forwarded to Administrative
Department Head Signature _____   Representative
                                         Date _____

Administrative Representative Comments:

_____

_____

_____

_____

_____

☐ Nomination Approved   Forwarded to C.A.R.E.
Corporate Staff Signature _____   Committee
                                         Date _____

C.A.R.E. Committee Comments:

_____

_____

_____

_____

_____

☐ Selected as C.A.R.E. Employee of the month for _____ _____ .
                                                  year

☐ Selected as C.A.R.E. Employee of the year _____ .

☐ Not Selected

CRITERIA FOR SELECTING C.A.R.E. EMPLOYEE OF THE MONTH

Supervisors are asked to nominate the employee who excels in the following behaviors in a given month. Final selections will also be based on the same criteria.

1. Acknowledges and greets visitors, patients and co-workers whenever s/he meets them.
2. Responds to patients, visitors and fellow-workers in a pleasant, respectful and professional way.
3. Anticipates the needs of visitors, patients and peers and helps them out whenever possible.
4. Introduces self, mentions his/her department or position, explains functions s/he is there to perform.
5. Answers the inquiries of patients, guests and co-workers (*especially new employees*) in a patient, helpful and positive way.
6. Obtains information or refers guests to proper source when unable to provide an answer.
7. Opens doors, holds open elevator doors for people wheeling carts or carrying things.
8. Practices listening and identifying skills when guests (*whether patient or visitor*) get upset.
9. Makes a special effort to practice CARE surface skills the first time s/he meets a patient, guest or co-worker.
10. Maintains a neat, well-groomed and professional appearance that creates a positive image for The Williamsport Hospital.
11. Does his/her part in helping to keep the hospital clean (*not leaving mess; picks up after self; picks up debris*).
12. Demonstrates concern for the rights, privacy and feelings of patients, guests and co-workers.
13. Interacts with others in a businesslike, professional manner; avoids idle conversation that excludes guests.
14. When time allows, answers phone this way:
    - (Greeting) Hello
    - (Department) eg. Maintenance
    - (Name Optional) John Moore (speaking)
    - (Climate Setter) May I help you?
15. Demonstrates concern for confidentiality of patient information when talking with the patient or when in public areas.
16. Treats hospital patients and visitors as guests to our "home".
17. Explains reasons for our rules, regulations and policies when asked to do so by patients and visitors.
18. Keeps his/her work environment neat and professional looking at all times.
19. Shows pride, interest and enthusiasm in his/her work.
20. Goes out of his/her way to recognize everyone s/he meets as an individual person.
21. Tries to be the kind of person others would like to work with.
22. Interacts with co-workers to help promote good working relationships.
23. Treats all employees regardless of department or position with dignity and respect.
24. Is in the habit of "helping out" fellow workers whenever s/he can.
25. Shows pride in The Williamsport Hospital (*together we are The Williamsport Hospital*).

Resource 6-B

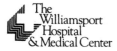
The Williamsport Hospital & Medical Center

C.A.R.E. PHYSICIAN NOMINATION

FROM:_____   _____
(Nominator/Nominators)   (Date)

_____   _____
(Department)   (Job Title)

TO: HUMAN RESOURCES DEPARTMENT

SUBJECT: C.A.R.E. Physician of the month Nomination.

I respectfully nominate:

_____
(Physician's Name)

for consideration as the C.A.R.E. Physician of the Month. The reasons for this nomination are:

_____
_____
_____
_____
_____
_____
_____
_____
_____
_____
_____
_____
_____
_____
_____
_____
_____
_____

(PLEASE COMPLETE IN BLACK INK)

PERS-2766 Rev. 11/92

293

A CQI System for Healthcare

PHYSICIAN OF THE MONTH NOMINATION

To assist you in your nomination for the C.A.R.E. Physician, please review the following questions and then summarize in narrative form in your nominating letter. The questions are not all inclusive; you may have additional reasons and justification for your nomination. These questions are intended to assist you in thinking about the physician's specific C.A.R.E. behaviors.

C.A.R.E. CRITERIA

How did this physician exhibit courtesy in his/her relationship with individual employees?

How did this physician demonstrate a positive attitude toward his/her work? In dealings with employees?

How did this physician demonstrate respect for employees? Did he/she treat them with dignity, concern?

How did this physician exhibit enthusiasm toward employees? Did he/she demonstrate a willingness to go out of the way to help them? Did he/she show pride in our Hospital?

Was the C.A.R.E. behavior described above a sustained effort over the month or an occasional incident?

Is your nomination of this physician based on feedback from others, your own observations, or both? please explain.

PERS-2766 (page 2) 11/92

Resource 6-C.
Chairman's Quality
Award—Fiscal Year
1993–94

Overview

In 1989 The Williamsport Hospital & Medical Center established The Chairman's Quality Award as a component of our commitment to excellence.

The Chairman's Quality Award program recognizes and rewards departments and their employees for outstanding quality efforts.

The objectives of the fiscal year 1993–94 award program is to:

- Provide initiative and direction to departmental quality-improvement efforts.
- Recognize outstanding quality-improvement achievements by departments.
- Communicate to the hospital family and community our quality-improvement accomplishments.
- Ensure continuous quality improvement and attention to our customers.

Our commitment to excellence is a commitment to continuously improve services to exceed customer expectations.

Time Line:

Project selection and approval	Approved Project Deadline	Sept. 30, 1993
Project CQI activity	Stage	Sept. 1993–Jan. 1994
Award submission	Deadline	Jan. 30, 1994
Award submissions— initial review and ranking	Stage	Feb. 1–15, 1994

Announcement of top five finalists for each category	Date	Feb. 16, 1994
Development of storyboards and displays	Stage	Feb. 16– Mar. 22, 1994
Quality fair	Date	March 24 and 25, 1994
Announcement of first place winners and grand winner	Date	March 24, 1994
Feedback summary reports	Stage	March–April 1994

Procedure:

1. All departments must identify at least one new key customer-oriented opportunity for improvement to be completed in fiscal year 1993–94.

   The opportunity must:
   A) Be in keeping with the corporate goals and objectives.
   B) Address a high-priority customer service or issue.
      *High priority— HI-RISK
      HI-COST
      HI-VOLUME
      CUSTOMER SATISFACTION
      and/or PROBLEM PRONE
   C) Address closing the gap between customer expectation and their perception of service delivery.
   D) Address any of the three dimensions of quality
      • C.A.R.E.
      • TQM
      • MEDIMPROVE

2. The project must be submitted to Bob Ireland on a completed CQI request form (attached) and approved by your corporate officer and the corporate staff.
3. Departments must undertake project activity and have reached the stage of quality-improvement recommendations, development of quality standards, and development of an implementation plan by mid-January 1994.
4. Quality award submissions must be submitted *in duplicate* to Bob Ireland by January 30, 1994.

    **Award submissions are limited to 25 pages in length. The submission should include at least those elements shown in the attached "Essentials Elements to Include in the award submission". If any elements do not apply to your project briefly explain why in the report.
5. Top five finalists in each CQI category should develop storyboards or displays for the quality fair March 24 and 25, 1994.

CQI Project Request

PROJECT TOPIC: _____ DATE: _____
Individual or group requesting: _____
Dimension of Quality: Priority:

❏ C.A.R.E.   ❏ High risk   ❏ High patient/family
❏ TQM Service Systems   ❏ High volume   satisfaction impact
❏ MEDIMPROVE   ❏ High cost   ❏ High physician
                          ❏ Problem prone   satisfaction impact

What process would this project address?   Is the process related to key customers   ❏ Yes   ❏ No   ❏ Unknown
Who are the customers the process impacts?
What part of the process should not be studied? Does this project address a clearly defined process that has easily identified start and end points?   ❏ Yes   ❏ No Does the project proposed describe an improvement opportunity, not a solution to be tried?   ❏ Yes   ❏ No
What perceived need led to your identification of this project?   Is this process currently being changed or scheduled for an overhaul in the near future?   ❏ Yes   ❏ No   ❏ Unknown

What data was collected or should be collected to verify the choice of this topic for focus?
What are the desired outcomes and anticipated changes as a result of this project?
What impact will this have on your customers? a)   Will that increase or decrease costs? Explain.
What work areas or specialties must be represented on the team to accomplish its mission?

Do all the managers concerned with this process agree that it is important to study and improve this process?	❑ Yes ❑ No ❑ Unknown
Are there enough managers, supervisors and employees willing to cooperate to make this work?	❑ Yes ❑ No ❑ Unknown

Is this process or aspects of it being studied by another group?   ❑ Yes   ❑ No   ❑ Unknown
How often and for how long do you estimate a team will need to meet to address this project?
Vice-president review: _____ Signature Recommendations: Date: _____

MEDIMPROVE Review: _____ Signature

C.A.R.E. Review _____ Signature

TQM Review _____ Signature

❑ Approved ❑ Disapproved

Recommendations:

Start Date: _____

Resource 6-D. 1993 Chairman's Quality Award

DEPARTMENTS	PROJECT TITLE	DIMENSION OF QUALITY	WORK AREAS INVOLVED	DESIRED OUTCOMES
Radiology/CT Scanning	Physicians/Patients Waiting	TQM/MEDIMPROVE	Technicians, Film File, Receptionist and Supervisors	Less repeats; reduced waiting time; increased satisfaction
Laboratory	Lab's Communication Process	TQM/MEDIMPROVE	All lab sections and Outpatient Lab	Reduced turn around time; increased productivity; cost containment
Nuclear Medicine	Consolidation of RIA & Clinical Laboratory	MEDIMPROVE	Chemistry Dept and RIA staff	Consolidation; improved testing availability; cost reduction
Heart and Lung Center	Recruitment of a Cardiovascular Surgery Physicians Assistant	MEDIMPROVE	ICU, CCU, OR, Cardiology MDs, Cardiac Surgeon	Increased availability to execute orders; enhanced post-op care
Heart and Lung Center Respiratory Therapy and Non-Invasive Cardiology	Maintenance Exercise Program (Pulmonary Patients)	TQM	Respiratory therapy and CHAMPS Staff	Improved overall program quality; reduce respiratory labor hours
Patient Transport Committee	Patient Transportation System Improvement	TQM	Mtl. Mgmt., Radiology, Rehab, Lab, Nursing, OR, ER, Heart & Lung	Reduced delivery time; increased service coverage; improved patient satisfaction; improved operations

DEPARTMENTS	PROJECT TITLE	DIMENSION OF QUALITY	WORK AREAS INVOLVED	DESIRED OUTCOMES
Maintenance and Environmental Services	Infectious Waste Disposal	TQM	Environmental Services; Maintenance	Reduced price; reduced liability; ease of handling
WorkCenter and Occupational Health	Occupational Health Service Delivery	TQM	Radiology, Lab, Billing, Family Practice, WorkCenter	Timely accurate scheduling; timely results information; clarified points of entry and responsibility
Sports Medicine	Improve Quality of Waiting Time for Patients and/or Family During Injury Clinics	C.A.R.E.	Receptionist, secretary, trainers, physical therapist, director	100% customer satisfaction; focus on needs and desires of patient or family
Home Health Skilled Care	Perinatal Home Care	MEDIMPROVE	Clinic, OB, Nursing, Home Health	tangible program; decrease high risk births; increased revenues
Home Health (Durable Medical Equipment)	Improve Customer Communication	C.A.R.E.	Telecommunications; Store staff; store mgmt.	timely & appropriate service to customer; improve staff productivity; improve service quality
Dietary	Patient Satisfaction with food	C.A.R.E./TQM	Dietary all areas, nursing units, maintenance	overall satisfaction 95%

DEPARTMENTS	PROJECT TITLE	DIMENSION OF QUALITY	WORK AREAS INVOLVED	DESIRED OUTCOMES
Cancer Services	Accessing O.P. Information for Quality Tumor Registry	TQM	Tumor registrar, MD office staff, OP Hem/Onc; Surgeons, Rad Oncologist	more consistent and accurate data available to MDs, Corporate Staff & Marketing
Environmental Services	Patient room total cleaning	TQM	Maintenance, nursing, envir. services	preventative maintenance; more productive; notification system for maintenance
Paramedic/ Emergency Departments	Improved Customers Satisfaction through personalized Communications	C.A.R.E.	Paramedic ED & Op staff. ER staff; WAAS staff	Improved interactions during waiting with patient and family; improve attentiveness
Operating Room and Anesthesia	OR Turn around time	MEDIMPROVE	OR staff; Anesthesia staff; OR Environmental Services	Comparison to national averages; specific time based on specialty; improved booking
Operating Room; Same Day; Endoscopy; Anesthesia	Same Day Services, Patient Waiting	TQM	Endoscopy, Same Day, OR, Anesthesia	Defined patient arrival time frame; decreased waiting time
Recovery Room	Nurse Patient Ratio/ Recovery Room— Alternative Transport as solution?	TQM/ MEDIMPROVE	Recovery Room; OR Nurse Assistants; OR	Increased nurse/patient ratio; cost efficiency

DEPARTMENTS	PROJECT TITLE	DIMENSION OF QUALITY	WORK AREAS INVOLVED	DESIRED OUTCOMES
Anesthesia	Anesthesia Preop process, Revisited	MEDIMPROVE	Medical Depts of Surgery & Anesthesia, Hospital Depts anesthesia & OR; PAT	Improved process and content of anesthesia workup; reduce lab work preop; cost controls
CCU/IMC & Heart & Lung Center	Angioplasty	MEDIMPROVE	IMC/CCU; Cath Lab; physicians; Nurses, 4 East	Increased customer satisfaction; new procedure
4 East; 3 East; 4 West; ICU	Patient Admission from ER to Units	TQM	ER, 4E, 3E, ICU, 4W	Patient transfer to room in acceptable time; appropriate report from ER to unit; preparation on unit; increased trust
Social Services	Accessing Quality Mental Health Care for Patients in Crisis	TQM	Social Services, ER staff & physicians, Medical director, Way Unit	Timely, customer-friendly, predictable pattern of support for patients requiring emergency mental health interventions
Ambulatory Care Clinic, Family Practice, Family Planning, BirthPlace	Healthy Beginnings Plus Program Improvements	TQM, C.A.R.E.	Family Planning; BirthPlace; Life Center; Ambulatory Care Clinic; Family Practice; Community Relations; Social Services	Increased volumes; greater patient satisfaction; increased awareness of services; improved infant care; improved patient environment

DEPARTMENTS	PROJECT TITLE	DIMENSION OF QUALITY	WORK AREAS INVOLVED	DESIRED OUTCOMES
Pharmacy Services	The Expedient Conversion of Intravenous Medications to the Least-Invasive Therapy	MEDIMPROVE	Pharmacy; Nursing; Gastroenterology; Infectious Disease	Eliminate delays in conversion; develop protocols for pharmacist and nurses; decreased cost
Pediatrics	Further Adaptation of CARE Behaviors to the Pediatric Patients and Family, Particularly the Culturally Diverse	C.A.R.E.	Pediatrics; Social Services	Staff understand child and family needs; better communication by C.A.R.E. behaviors
Way Unit & Social Services	Integrated Discharge Planning	MEDIMPROVE	Nursing; Social Services	Earlier planning; increased patient participation and satisfaction
4 North	Cancer Pain Management	MEDIMPROVE	PCM, CN IV, & staff nurse, LPN, MD, Clinical Pharmacology	Promote pain management as patient right and professional responsibility; adherence to standards
3 West	Orientation to Rehab Video	TQM; MEDIMPROVE	All Rehab Disciplines	Improved retention of information about routines; increased patient participation in therapies; cost-effective use of nurses' time

DEPARTMENTS	PROJECT TITLE	DIMENSION OF QUALITY	WORK AREAS INVOLVED	DESIRED OUTCOMES
BirthPlace	Mother—Baby Nursing	TQM; MEDIMPROVE	Drs. Lamade, Odorizzi, Wetstone; Rosalie, Ami Jones, Cathy Kordes	Increase patient and family satisfaction; increased efficiency and productivity; improved patient education
Volunteer Services	Gift Box Customer Service	C.A.R.E./TQM	Volunteer Dept; Gift Box volunteers; Auxiliary Gift Box committee; employee representatives	Increased customer satisfaction
Management Engineering; CQI Tools Team	CQI Tools Training & CQI Facilitator training	TQM	CQI Tools Team	CQI reference manual; cadre of trained facilitator; departmental CQI training program
Volunteer Services	Information Center; Response to Reduction of Staff Hours	TQM	Info center staff; Supervisor; Assistant director Volunteers; Director Community Affairs	Volunteers/TEEN trained & increased confidence in ability; staff commit themselves
Marketing/ Community Relations	"How to Packet" for our clients	TQM	Marketing and Community Relations	Documented customer satisfaction levels; communication materials and marketing needs viewed as essential part business plans

DEPARTMENTS	PROJECT TITLE	DIMENSION OF QUALITY	WORK AREAS INVOLVED	DESIRED OUTCOMES
LifeCenter	Cholesterol Identification, Awareness and Education	MEDIMPROVE	Community services staff; health educators; phlebotomist, volunteers, and marketing	Increased awareness, educations and identification of cholesterol; improved screening; improved quality of life for customers
Admissions/ Utilization Review	One call scheduling	TQM	OR; Admissions, Utilization Review	Central Scheduling of OR cases; Pre-registration of patients prior to arrival; certification of medical necessity
Quality Assessment & Medical Records, Risk Management	MedisGroup Abstacting Incentive Program	MEDIMPROVE	Risk Mgr; Director Health Records; QA Supervisor	Reduced backlog of records needing review; improved employee morale and motivation; re-institute MedisGroup data for Medical Staff
MIS; Fiscal Svcs; Human Resources	Increased Time Management Productivity	TQM	MIS, Fiscal Svcs, Human Resources, Nursing	Implementation of an automated time and attendance system; increased accountability and productivity of labor cost

DEPARTMENTS	PROJECT TITLE	DIMENSION OF QUALITY	WORK AREAS INVOLVED	DESIRED OUTCOMES
Psychology Services	Diagnostic/ Psychotherapy Case Conference	MEDIMPROVE	Psychology staff; Medical staff; Social Services	Increased knowledge across a wider range of diagnostic and treatment techniques; reduction in stress in staff
Telecommunica- tions and Fiscal Services	Better Management of Patient Inquiry Call Loads to the Business Office	TQM	Fiscal Services staff; Telecommunications staff	Improved call-management and patient interactions during walk-in visits
Chaplaincy Services	Chaplaincy Care Competencies	C.A.R.E.	CPE students, Chaplain volunteer visitors; Chaplain on-call volunteers	High level of respect expressed for patient and family beliefs; timeliness of chaplain visits
Learning Resources	Wayfinding	TQM	Sign Committee; Maintenance; Marketing; Nursing	wayfinding much easier for customers
H.R. Gibson Rehab.	Patient Concerns/Complaints	C.A.R.E.	Rehab clinician; nursing; social Svcs; administration; consumer	Increased satisfaction; improved communication with patients

DEPARTMENTS	PROJECT TITLE	DIMENSION OF QUALITY	WORK AREAS INVOLVED	DESIRED OUTCOMES
H.R. Gibson Rehab.	First Day Therapy— 3 West Admissions	MEDIMPROVE	Rehab clinicians, nursing, Rehab coordinator, Case. Mgr., physician	No less than 1 hour of therapy on 1st day; specific instructions for nursing dept re. ambulation & ADL activities
Health Education Research foundation	Review and Revise Physician Billing System	TQM	all HERF Offices; Physician Practice Admin.; MIS—PBS support staff	Enhancement to patient service; improvement to staff productivity
Infection Control	Tuberculosis Control	MEDIMPROVE	Maintenance; Employee Health; Nursing; Endoscopy; SDS; Respiratory; Radiology; ER; Paramedics; Admissions; MD office representative	Be in compliance with 1990 CDC guidelines; provide a safe environment

INDEX

228–29
Dietrich, Joanne, 153
Divine Providence Hospital, SHS
alliance, 207–33
Doctors. *See* Physicians
Donabedian, Avedis, 198
Downey, Chris, 146
DPH. *See* Divine Providence
Hospital
Draper, Elizabeth A., 202
DRGs. *See* Diagnostic related groups
Drucker, Peter, 12, 88

Emergency room, 7, 43
Employees
awards. *See* Recognition and
rewards
C.A.R.E. behaviors, 60–63,
93–96
certification, 173, 182–85
communication with, 41, 74–77
customer relations, 40, 89; *See
also* Magic moments;
Moments of truth
difficult, 106–10, 162–63
empowering, 88, 136–44
firing, 58, 80–83, 163, 190
hiring, 117, 173, 174–75, 180–85,
190
lay–offs, 80–83
manager relations, 15–16, 41, 89,
162–63, 178–80
morale, 80, 166–71, 192–93, 225
motivation of, 70–74, 153–56,
190, 261–64
performance evaluation, 59–60,
156–60, 251–60
quality pursuit and, 26–27, 28,
168–69, 198–99
recognition. *See* Recognition and
rewards

treatment of, 14–15, 41, 105–106,
178–80
English, Joseph, 50, 60, 172
Epic Healthcare Group, 167–68
Equity theory, 73, 263
Evans, Donnie, 153
Expectancy theory, 74, 262–63

Facilitators, 101–5
Factor price equalization, 17
Federal Express, 2
Feedback, 60, 157, 159, 196–98,
253
Finn, Marcia, 29, 50
Finnigan, Jerome P., 3
Firing, 58, 80–83, 163, 190
Fisher, Dean, 29
Frailey, Gregory, 50
Frankl, Viktor E., 70

Geedey, Nancy, 153
Geeneen, Harold, 18
Givens, Charles J., 203
Glunk, Dan, 50
Go–Beyond Quality Outcome, 86
Go–beyond service, 8–10, 155
Goodman, Ellen, 10
Grace, Mark, 15
Green, Paul, 181
Gulledge, Keith, 23, 167

Hall, Robert, 205
Head to Head (Thurow), 17
Healthcare
costs, 17, 93–95
CQI implementation, 1–22,
207–33
managed care, 227–29
strategic planning need, 20–22
Healthcare Forum, viii, xvii
Heiney, Dave, 177, 180